the food coach

Judy Davie coaches people to enjoy the benefits of eating healthier food. Her interest in macrobiotic cooking and food as medicine led to her involvement in the popular television show *Search for a Supermodel* before she founded her company, The Food Coach, in 2001. She presents to organisations on the value of food, writes a column for *Woman's Day*, and features regularly on ABC Radio, Sydney. She moved to Australia from Scotland in 1986 after studying biology, psychology and health and exercise.

www.thefoodcoach.com.au

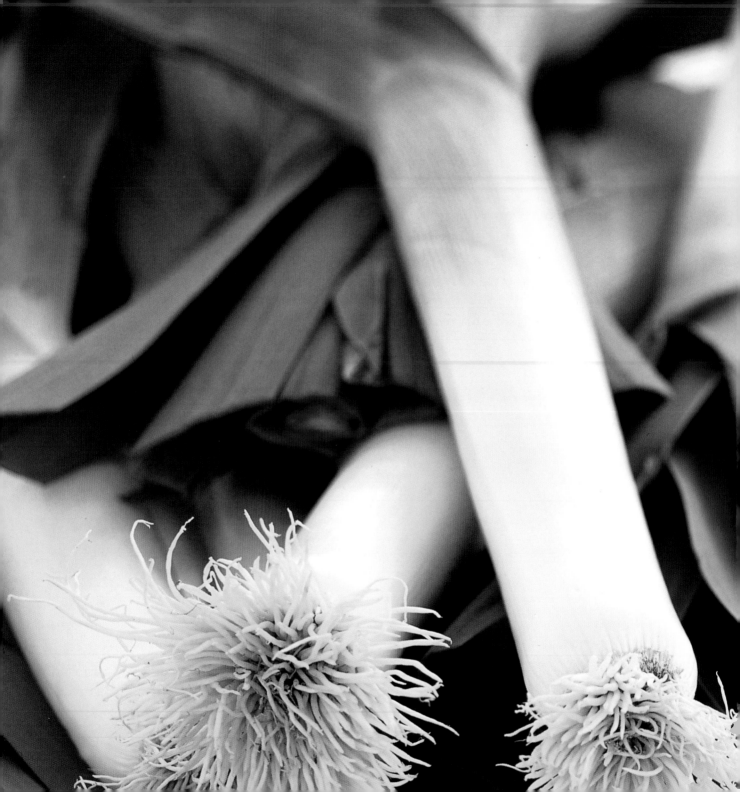

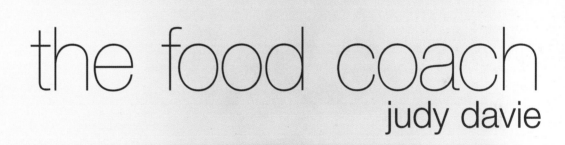

the food coach

judy davie

photography by john paul urizar

VIKING
an imprint of
PENGUIN BOOKS

This book is dedicated to my mother, Biddy, who brought me up to be healthy and strong and who allowed me to spread my wings and make a life for myself.

Viking

Penguin Group (Australia)
250 Camberwell Road, Camberwell, Victoria 3124, Australia
Penguin Books Ltd
80 Strand, London WC2R 0RL, England
Penguin Group (USA) Inc.
375 Hudson Street, New York, New York 10014, USA
Penguin Books, a division of Pearson Canada
10 Alcorn Avenue, Toronto, Ontario, Canada M4V 3B2
Penguin Books (NZ) Ltd
Cnr Rosedale and Airborne Roads, Albany, Auckland, New Zealand
Penguin Books (South Africa) (Pty) Ltd
24 Sturdee Avenue, Rosebank, Johannesburg 2196, South Africa
Penguin Books India (P) Ltd
11, Community Centre, Panchsheel Park, New Delhi 110 017, India

First published by Penguin Group (Australia), a division of Pearson Australia Group Pty Ltd, 2004

10 9 8 7 6 5 4 3 2 1

Cover and text design by Melissa Fraser © Penguin Group (Australia)
Styling by Julz Beresford
Cover photograph by John Paul Urizar
Typeset in Bembo by Post Pre-press Group, Brisbane Queensland
Printed and bound in China by Imago Productions

National Library of Australia
Cataloguing-in-Publication data:

    Davie, Judy, 1962– .
    The food coach.

    Includes index.
    ISBN 0 670 04115 7.

    1. Cookery. 2. Quick and easy cookery. I. Urizar, John
    Paul. II. Title.

641.555

www.penguin.com.au

contents

preface

Ten years ago my mother and I travelled to Honolulu. For her it was a trip down memory lane from forty-five years earlier. Few places were the same but the old crumbling hotel where she and my grandparents once stayed was still there. It was in that hotel in 1949 that she tried her first Coca-Cola.

I remember my first McDonald's burger, twenty years ago, but I have no memory of when I first tried a beautiful ripe avocado, mango, or any of the food nature provides. It's alarming that many of the things we consume so readily were not in existence fifty years ago, yet these foods are so heavily marketed, they are now more widely accepted and consumed than natural food that has been around for centuries.

My love of food started as a child. I loved it so much that my father nicknamed me 'Jude the Pude', 'Poodie', and other derivatives of the word 'pudding'. It was less about being fat and more about the quantity I ate. I loved pudding, bread, savouries, sweets, salads, roasts, anything and everything (except tripe and liver). Rather than being told to finish everything on the plate, I was told to stop racing through my meal in the hope I could have more. Despite the large quantities I ate, I was solid but not the proportions of the barrage balloon you might be imagining right now.

My mother enjoyed cooking and virtually everything we ate came from her kitchen: breads, biscuits, oatcakes, soups, casseroles, cakes, pies, the lot. We ate sweets on Sundays as a special treat and were never denied anything from the cupboard. Mum cooked with a variety of grains, including oats, barley and rice; the butcher delivered meat and eggs most days; and we had fish on Fridays. In the winter months we had mandarins, apples and pears, and in summer luscious strawberries and peaches followed by late-season raspberries. The vegetables available were carrots, broccoli, potatoes, Brussels sprouts, peas and, on very special occasions, asparagus.

When I left home for the first time it was my love of good food that steered me into the kitchen to learn for myself how to prepare a good meal. I never considered buying anything in a packet, so I started with eggs and cabbage and bit by bit gained the confidence to play with other ingredients. After many years of experimenting in the kitchen, dieting, and studying macrobiotic cooking and food as medicine, I have no doubt that we should approach food with a greater purpose other than merely to satisfy hunger.

My upbringing is a testimony to the fact that healthy food can be delicious. I have my mother to thank for my strong constitution, as I am certain that the food she fed me built the solid foundation of my being.

In this book I use ingredients from my youth combined in new and interesting ways. My collection of recipes will lead you to improved health as you discover that healthy food is not only quick and easy to prepare but also delicious.

introduction

When people ask me what a food coach is, I tell them it's a **personal trainer in healthy eating.** A food coach trains people to recognise that food does more than just fill a gap, make you fat or help you stay slim. Food coaching helps people recognise that the food they choose to eat affects how they feel. By knowing what food does for your body, you can select food that will make you feel better than you thought possible. It's also about loving food and enjoying eating. As a food coach, I train people to eat healthier food than they would normally. I help them to focus on how much better they feel when they eat well. I encourage them to get back into the kitchen and prepare quick, easy and delicious healthy meals. I hope that this book will help you to do the same.

If there were six dishes to choose from and you liked all of them, wouldn't it make the most sense to choose the one that you not only liked, but would also do your body the most good? That's the key to leading a healthy life through food. It's not about sacrifice, denial and body image. It's about **freedom, flexibility, fun and feeling great!** When you feel great, life's great and by default . . . guess what? You look great.

When I started food coaching, I realised that it wasn't enough to tell people what they should eat and why. Many people today need help with the 'how'. Although less time is spent in the kitchen than in years gone by, I would argue that as much time can be spent heating up food that is not so good for you as in cooking food that is. The trick with food coaching is to teach people how to prepare healthy food quickly. I started by creating some recipes that I refer to as 'gate to plate' recipes – fast, easy meals that can be whipped up in less time than it would take to heat a frozen pie in the microwave (I shudder at the thought!). After 'auditing' my clients' pantries to get rid of unhealthy items, we create a shopping list and head off to the health food shop, greengrocer and supermarket to stock up on new ingredients. A few cooking sessions later, many ingredients once considered weird and unfamiliar have become commonplace.

I also created a 'toolkit' of recipes – basic ingredients and greens around which my clients could build a meal. Once you have the toolkit ingredients on hand, you can create **delicious meals in a flash**.

The emphasis with food coaching must always be on 'healthier' eating – eating better than you normally would and noticing how much better you feel as a result. This book therefore provides recipes for everyone. There are recipes for meat eaters and for the most health-conscious, recipes with no sugar or butter and very little cheese. All flours and grains used are whole grains, and many of the meals are designed around a cooked green vegetable or salad. Even if you do nothing else but resolve always to serve some green vegetables or salad with the evening meal, you'll be well on the way to better health.

If you feel a little daunted by the prospect of conquering the kitchen, take comfort in the knowledge that I am not a great master chef. I am a good cook now, but I wasn't always. I like to eat, I love being healthy, and, now that I am over forty, I really love people telling me that I look younger than my years! If you like the sound of that, then you are more than halfway there already.

The Food Coach is a collection of recipes that are nutritious and taste great. I hope it helps you get into the habit of eating well all the time.

the value of food

I categorise food very simply, into value-positive and value-negative – that is, food that will do your body good and food that won't.

'Value-positive food' provides the body with all it needs to perform normal bodily functions well. It is fuel that the body burns cleanly and efficiently, with the resulting waste products passed out of the body quickly. A body fuelled with value-positive food is glowing, vital, youthful, lean and full of energy. (See the Glossary of value-positive foods on pages 176–80 for more information.)

'Value-negative food', however, burdens the body. The energy expended to process this food is energy that could be put to better use elsewhere – to work and play and think. Value negative food can be stored as fat and may cause the build-up of toxins in the body, causing a range of imbalances and effects, including mood swings, fatigue, skin conditions, allergies, obesity, high blood pressure, heart disease, stress, diabetes and cancer.

Without getting too technical, the body uses food as fuel, to propel and drive all the systems in the body efficiently. From food the body also draws the nutrients it needs to perform these tasks as effectively as possible. Food goes in the mouth, where the digestive process starts. During digestion the body takes what it needs, breaking down the food into usable components and sending these off to where they are needed. Once this is done, the remainder of the food is passed out of the body – in an ideal world that is.

In our less ideal world, some foods don't provide exactly what the body wants and some don't pass through as quickly as they should. Foods lacking in nutrients and foods that are not digested completely can slow us down, and create toxic build-up and fat. Maybe the simplest way to explain it is just to say that the body is not man-made and therefore the food we eat shouldn't be either. A diet of fresh produce, in season, is the key to good health.

Buy your food as fresh as possible and minimise foods from boxes or cans. Get into the habit of reading labels and select the brands with the lowest amounts of sodium and sugar, preservatives, colourings and other additives.

If you eat meat, try to buy organic. It might cost more, but believe me you'll notice the difference. Aside from being free of pesticides and artificial hormones, it tastes better. Some people refer to 'prana' – energy or life force – in food. I am certain that the meat from an animal will always taste better if it has led a happy and healthy life.

Not so long ago we were told to eat a low-fat diet and the food industry responded by producing low-fat everything. Biscuits, cakes, drinks, dairy products, breakfast bars – you name it. But most of these low-fat products were incredibly high in carbohydrates. Today we are told to eat a diet low in carbohydrates and high in protein. The food industry is now responding by making protein bars and powders, but these are just more processed foods. Our nation got fatter with the low-fat regime; it will be interesting to see what happens to us in the protein phase.

As well as keeping away from processed foods as much as possible, you should also consider the GI value of the food you eat. The GI (glycaemic index) is a measure of the speed at which the body converts carbohydrates into glucose. The body converts all carbohydrates into glucose for energy, but foods with a high GI are converted quickly for an almost instant fix but no sustained energy, while foods with a low GI will provide energy for a much longer period.

As much as possible, you should avoid trans fatty acids. These are produced during the processing of refined oils, when unsaturated fatty acids are exposed to heat and light or are hydrogenated. They are found in margarines and in prepared biscuits, cakes and the like. Trans fatty acids increase cholesterol levels in the body, can damage the immune system and may promote heart disease and cancer. Buy cold-pressed, extra-virgin olive oil and look out for table spreads that do not contain hydrogenated fats. Omega-3 fatty acids, on the other hand, strengthen the immune system and cleanse the heart and arteries. They are found in fish, linseeds and many other healthy foods. When the recipes in this book call for 'olive oil', you should use cold-pressed, extra-virgin olive oil.

measurements

One of the biggest bores for reluctant cooks is all the weighing and measuring required to produce a decent meal. We often see great chefs at work on TV who seem to be using quite a bit of licence when it comes to adding ingredients: 'A handful of this and a splash of that.' This requires the kind of confidence gained only from experience. Until that confidence comes, I find measuring in cups and spoons much easier and quicker than dragging out the kitchen scales and measuring jugs, so most of the ingredients in these recipes are measured using cups and spoons.

On the other hand, you need to know what weight of meat and fish to buy. I generally work on 125 g (4 oz) per adult serve, unless it is being mixed with vegetables, for example in kebabs or stir-fries, when you will only need half this amount.

If you prefer to work with more precise measurements, this table provides the approximate equivalents in millilitres and fluid ounces.

1 cup	½ cup	⅓ cup	¼ cup	1 tablespoon	1 teaspoon
250 ml (8 fl oz)	125 ml (4 fl oz)	80 ml (2½ fl oz)	60 ml (2 fl oz)	20 ml (⅔ fl oz)	5 ml (⅙ fl oz)

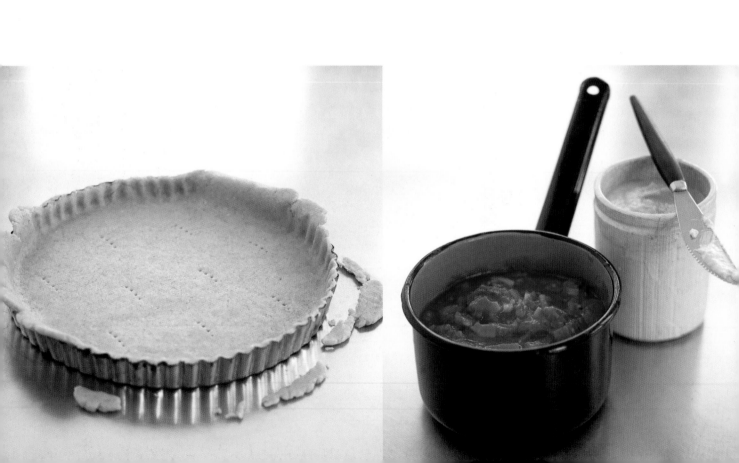

your toolkit

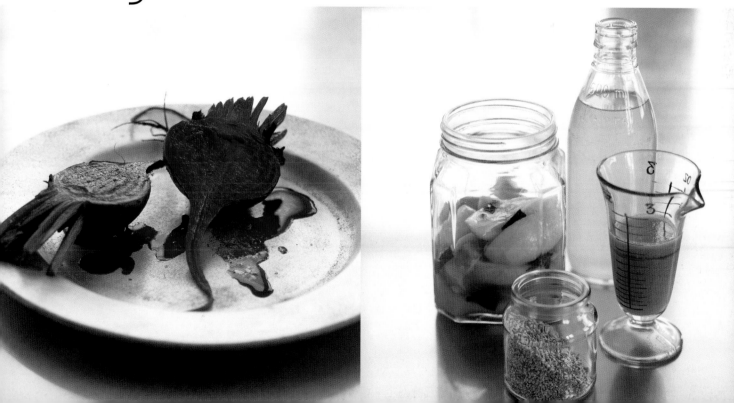

I sometimes use a fashion analogy when describing my style of cooking. Take a good suit or a little black dress and you can create many different looks simply by changing your accessories. A change of belt or tie or jewellery can transform the same outfit over and over again. With healthy eating, the same rules apply: a basic recipe can be used to transform many different ingredients and make many different dishes. I call it my recipe toolkit.

A batch of hummus made on the weekend can be served with Middle Eastern mezze in the evening, on sandwiches at lunch or under a piece of fish for dinner at night. Dashi forms the basis of many exciting Japanese dishes, and za'tar, a very simple spice mix, can be used to create the most exotic dishes.

The recipes in this book show you how to use the toolkit in simple, tasty ways. But these are just a few of many delicious combinations that can be created using the toolkit. Using them should encourage you to experiment with flavours and combinations yourself. There is no *right* way to cook great food – if the ingredients are healthy and taste good together, go for it!

Whatever you cook, eat lots of vegetables, especially the GLVs (green leafy vegetables). I am definitely an 'eat your greens' fanatic! My mission is to convert those who shudder at the thought of anything green to the delights of these nutritionally marvellous foods. I hope to inspire you with recipes that will make you want to load your fridge and plate with GLVs. Make greens the focus of your meal and plant other yummy things around your plate.

If you are still not convinced, maybe this will persuade you. Vegetables contain abundant amounts of anti-oxidants, which fight free radicals (molecules that destroy cells in the body). The bottom line is that, amongst other things, GLVs help you battle ageing.

Always wash your leaves – I'd hate you to be put off GLVs by finding a slug on your plate – and use this little trick from my macrobiotic teacher, Karla Maverick, who called it 'energetically' cutting them. Fold the leaves in half lengthwise. Using a sharp knife, cut in the same direction as the veins of the leaf. Cut the stalk lengthwise (this retains the life force of the plant, providing a greater source of energy for those eating the vegetable – and, incredibly enough, makes the vegetable taste more delicious).

 Whenever you see this icon in an ingredients list, it indicates that the ingredient comes from my recipe toolkit or green leafy vegetables.

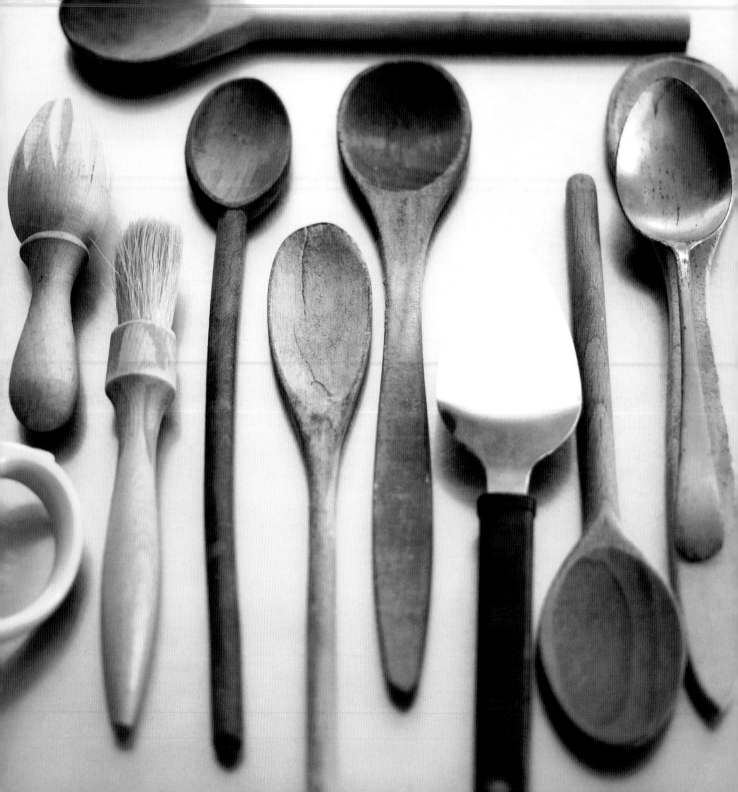

BASIC UTENSILS

There are a number of pieces of kitchen equipment that will help you prepare food quickly and efficiently in our time-poor society. You don't have to fill your kitchen with all the tools of a master chef, but without some basic pieces of equipment it can be too hard. A good knife can reduce preparation time by half, likewise a garlic press. Conversely, don't be fooled into buying every gadget ever made, as many will only cost you time in assembly and washing up, and take up valuable shelf space.

When compiling this list I kept in mind someone who is setting up their kitchen for the first time. It contains everything I use regularly and would hate to be without.

baking trays One large, one medium and one or two baking sheets.

bamboo steamers Two sizes – small and large.

casserole dish Useful for winter dishes.

chargrill (barbecue) pan Very useful if you live in a unit and don't have a barbecue. Make sure you have the extractor fan switched on during grilling or your home will fill with smoke and you may end up with the fire brigade outside your door.

chopping board Two is preferable – one for meat and fish, the other for fruit and vegetables.

colander and fine sieve One of these is an absolute must – both are better still.

food processor If my house was burning down I'd grab my photos, paintings and food processor – everyone should have one.

frying pan Large, with a lid.

garlic press Saves time.

grater Get a multi-sided one.

knives Never compromise on the quality of your knives. Once you have used a good-quality knife, you will never want to cook with anything of a lower standard again. With a well-balanced blade, food preparation is quicker, the food tastes better and there's less chance of injuring yourself.

ladle Not essential, but it beats scooping soup out of a pan with a cup!

loaf tin When you feel like making something sweet and comforting you'll need this to make a healthy alternative.

measuring spoons and cups Up there with the food processor.

metal hand whisk For egg whites.

mini-muffin tray See loaf tin.

mortar and pestle or spice grinder You'll need this to grind your spices after you've roasted them.

pastry brush You should use this often, to ensure that you don't overdo the oil.

pepper grinder Commercially ground pepper is an irritant; freshly ground pepper has many healthy properties and tastes much better too.

salad spinner I salute the creator of this nifty piece of equipment. Gone are the days of waving around wet lettuce wrapped in a tea towel or of eating slugs.

scissors Try to store them in the same place at all times. Mine always go missing whenever I need them!

slotted spoon A very handy tool for poaching fish and eggs and serving chunky sauces.

slow cooker Most useful in winter for making soups and porridges.

small non-stick omelette or pancake pan You will probably be surprised how often you use this. Mine is often dug out if I want to throw together a quick omelette mid-week, or to roast seeds and spices quickly.

spatula Can't do without this.

stainless-steel mixing bowls Small, medium and large – for a myriad of uses.

stainless-steel saucepans Invest in good-quality pans – they will last a lifetime. A good starting kit is one large stockpot (great for making soup), one 20 cm (8 in) pan, one 15 cm (6 in) pan and one small milk pan.

sushi mat Other than its obvious use, this is good for squeezing excess moisture from spinach.

tongs Every kitchen must have at least one pair of tongs.

vegetable peeler Much better than a sharp knife and great for making vegetable chips.

wire cake rack For cooling baked biscuits and cakes.

wok This is a mid-week 'must-have'. So many delicious and healthy meals can be created in a wok in no time at all.

wooden hand-held lemon juicer Much handier than electric juicers.

wooden spoons Worth having two.

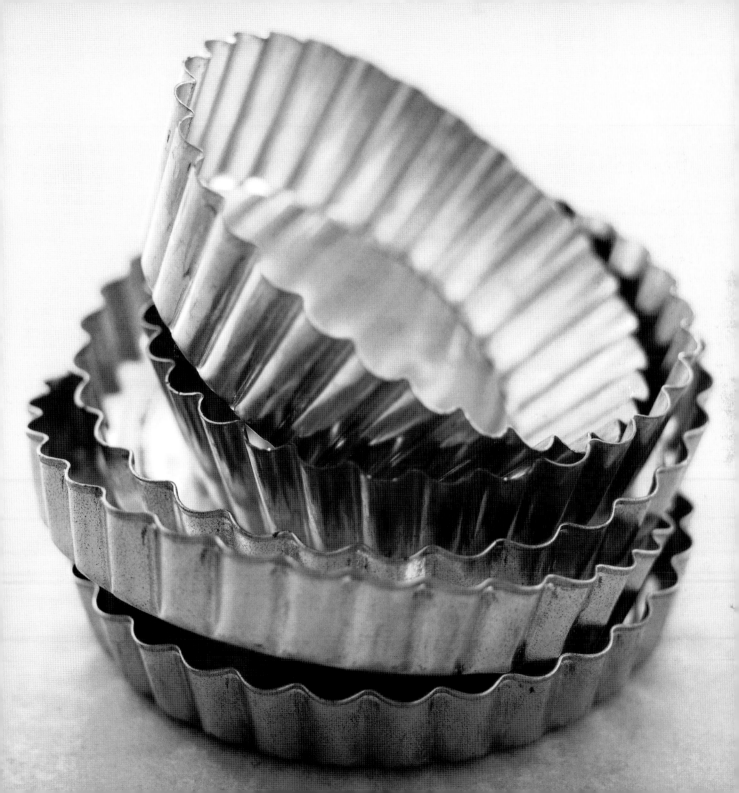

ESSENTIAL PANTRY

Are you brave enough to venture into your pantry and sort it out? Why not dedicate a couple of hours to the task? Start by throwing out all the jars of things that are out of date. Pay particular attention to any oils that are old – they can become rancid, and are particularly damaging to your health. Once the out-of-date foods are in the bin, consider throwing out any items that have been lurking in the cupboard in open containers and plastic packets. Chances are you won't be eating them again, either.

Now that you're feeling virtuous, you can move on to checking the labels on the remaining packages. Check for preservatives, flavourings and colouring additives then decide what to keep and what to throw out. If your cupboards are left bare, here's a list of essential items to keep in your pantry that will help you make delicious, healthy meals in record-breaking time.

pantry

cold-pressed, extra-virgin olive oil

corn oil

sesame oil

walnut oil

balsamic vinegar

brown rice vinegar

fish sauce

raw almonds

slivered almonds

pine nuts

walnuts

buckwheat flour

kudzu or cornflour (cornstarch)

organic wholemeal plain (all-purpose) flour

organic wholemeal self-raising (self-rising) flour

buckwheat noodles

couscous

polenta (cornmeal)

chickpeas (garbanzo beans) – dried or organic canned

haricot (navy) beans – dried or organic canned

kidney beans – dried or organic canned

organic canned peeled tomatoes

kombu

bonito flakes

apple concentrate

honey

maple syrup

pear concentrate

rice syrup

cumin seeds

nigella seeds (sometimes called black cumin seeds)

dried marjoram

dried thyme

sumac

black pepper

sea salt

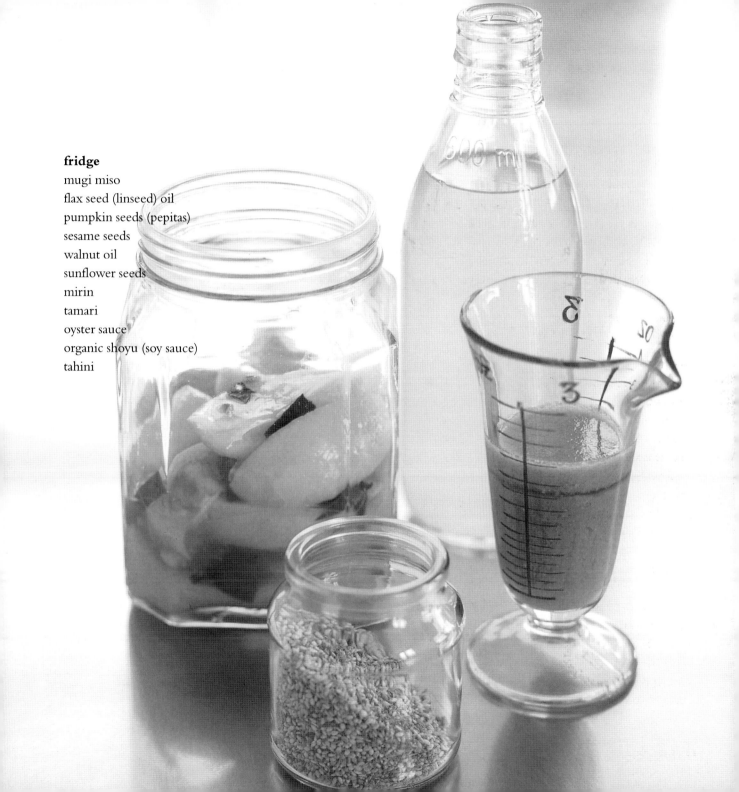

fridge

mugi miso

flax seed (linseed) oil

pumpkin seeds (pepitas)

sesame seeds

walnut oil

sunflower seeds

mirin

tamari

oyster sauce

organic shoyu (soy sauce)

tahini

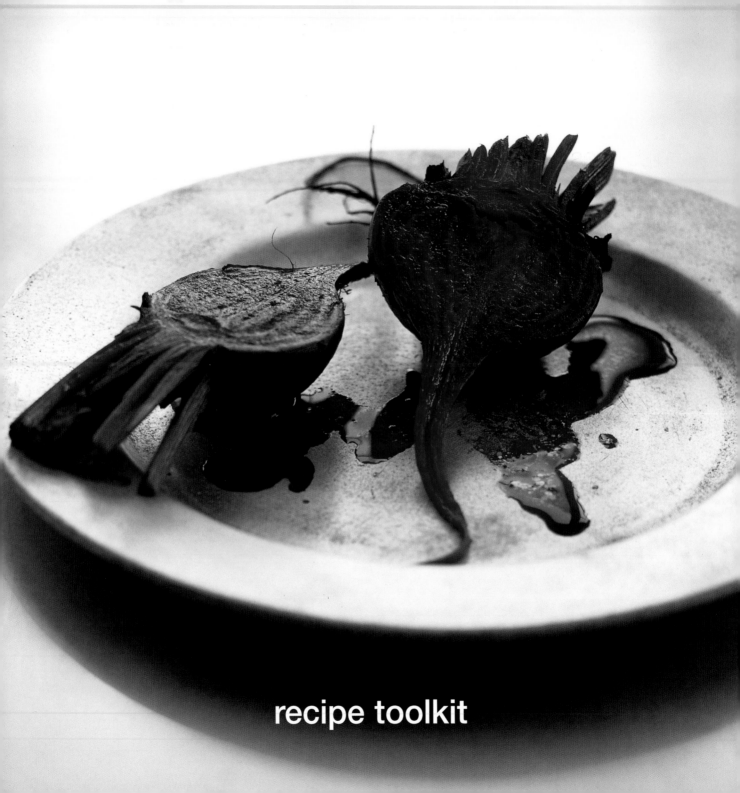

recipe toolkit

miso dressing

This dressing is a great base for a variety of dishes. I was introduced to it by Karla Maverick, my macrobiotic cooking teacher. Karla used this recipe in a dish with pinto beans but I have found many uses for it and now pull it from the toolkit regularly. Pour it over a winter salad of grated red cabbage, apple, carrots and onion, or use it to flavour baked fish. It's used in a few of my favourite recipes in this book, but don't limit yourself to the list below. I've said it before – never be afraid to experiment.

1 tablespoon mugi miso
1 tablespoon olive oil
2 tablespoons brown rice vinegar
3 tablespoons water

makes about ½ cup

Combine the miso and oil in a small bowl and mix thoroughly. Add the vinegar and water separately, mixing thoroughly after each addition. The dressing will keep for up to 6 weeks in the fridge.

Use miso dressing in
• white bean and dill dip (page 54)
• buckwheat noodle, bok choy and pine nut salad (page 84)
• avocado and bean salad (page 89)
• baked ocean trout with bean mash and Asian greens (page 124)

za'tar

I first stumbled upon za'tar in a Middle Eastern spice stand at the Byron Bay markets one Sunday. It's so exciting when you discover a new taste that you know will complement a multitude of delicious dishes.

If you live in the city, you will no doubt find a shop that sells ready-made za'tar, but don't despair if you can't – it's easy to make your own. Once you've tried it, I'm sure you'll always have a jar around.

3 tablespoons sesame seeds

1 tablespoon finely grated lemon zest

4 heaped teaspoons dried thyme

2 heaped teaspoons dried marjoram

2 heaped teaspoons sumac (or 1 level teaspoon sea salt)

makes 6 tablespoons

Dry-roast the sesame seeds and lemon zest in a heavy-based pan over a low heat for about 6 minutes or until the seeds darken and become fragrant and the zest dries out. Grind the thyme and marjoram to a powder using a mortar and pestle or spice grinder. Mix the powder through the sesame seed and lemon zest mixture, along with the sumac or sea salt. You can make large batches of this spice mix and store it in an airtight container in the fridge.

Use za'tar in

- Middle Eastern mezze (page 51)
- rocket, basil and avocado salad with nigella seeds (page 96)
- chargrilled ocean perch and kumara mash (page 138)
- lemon za'tar chicken with chargrilled zucchini and spinach (page 150)

preserved lemons

My first two weeks in Australia were spent at my cousin Neil's house in Perth. It was mid-January and his lemon tree was weighed down with fruit. I'd never seen lemons on a tree before; my only point of reference were the lemons in UK supermarkets. Cousin Neil's wife, Julie, was somewhat bewildered when I scooped the lemons off the ground and pored over her recipe books looking for 101 things to do with a lemon. I wish I had stumbled on a recipe for preserved lemons then, but in those days I hadn't been exposed to Middle Eastern cuisine. Perhaps Australia hadn't either back in 1986.

Preserved lemons are now an essential item in my recipe toolkit. They pep up grilled (broiled) fish, roast vegetables and grains, among other things. You can buy them, or make your own. The recipe here is very easy and you can ensure the quality by using sea salt. They are *very* salty, so do use them in moderation and eat only the peel.

The number of lemons in the recipe is a suggestion only. Their size and the amount of juice they yield will determine how many you need to fill the jars. Lemons with thicker skins are the best.

4 x 500 ml (16 fl oz) jars with secure lids
1 cup sea salt
24 lemons
4 x 2.5 cm (1 in) pieces cassia bark
4 bay leaves
8 whole peppercorns

makes 4 jars

Thoroughly wash the jars. To dry and sterilise them, place on a baking tray in the oven at a very low heat (120°C, 250°F, Gas Mark 1) for 5–7 minutes. Place 2 teaspoons of the salt into each jar. Select 12 of the most unblemished lemons and scrub them to remove their waxy coating. Squeeze the juice from the remaining lemons into a jug, straining off the pips and pulp. Put the remaining salt into a large bowl. Cut the 12 scrubbed lemons into quarters lengthways and place them in the bowl of salt, rubbing the salt into them with your hands. Pack the lemons into the jars, skin-side facing down, and fill each jar with the lemon juice, ensuring that the lemons are completely covered. Distribute the cassia bark, bay leaves and peppercorns evenly among the jars and fasten the lids. Store the jars in a cool cupboard and up-end them each week so that half the time they are standing on their lids. The lemons will be ready to eat in 6–8 weeks, when the skin is soft. Once opened, store the jar in the fridge for up to 6 months. Unopened jars will keep for up to 6 months in the pantry.

Use preserved lemons in
• Moroccan couscous (page 66)
• root vegetable salad (page 94)
• baked mackerel (page 131)
• baked snapper (page 132)
• moonfish with cucumber and lemon salsa (page 142)

hummus

We all have a recipe for hummus and most corner shops sell it in tubs, but making your own is easy and I think this version tastes much better than any of the shop brands.

Think outside the square when it comes to serving hummus. It is a lovely dip with crudités and crackers, but it's also delicious under grilled fish, as an alternative to mash, as a filling for miniature savoury flans or served with other beans as a healthier substitute for sour cream.

1 can organic chickpeas (garbanzo beans)
1 large clove Russian garlic (or 3 cloves ordinary garlic)
¼ cup tahini
juice of 1 lemon (or 2 limes)
1 teaspoon chilli oil
¼ cup olive oil
cracked black pepper, to taste

makes 1½ cups

Drain the chickpeas, reserving 3 tablespoons of water from the can. Put the chickpeas and reserved water in a food processor and process until smooth. Add the garlic, tahini and lemon juice and continue to process. With the processor running, add the chilli oil and then slowly pour in the olive oil. Process, process, process – and when you think you have processed enough, do it some more. The hummus will lighten in colour and turn really creamy. Add pepper to taste. Hummus will keep in the fridge for up to 7 days.

Use hummus in
- Middle Eastern mezze (page 51)
- grilled tuna and beans with chilli-limed hummus and slow-roasted tomatoes (page 127)

dashi

Most people believe Japanese food is very healthy, but when you go exploring Japanese and Korean supermarkets you will find that they too have an enormous range of packaged products, many containing monosodium glutamate and lots of other additives and preservatives. Traditional Japanese cuisine, like traditional cuisines all over the world, works with a few main ingredients. Dashi (stock), shoyu (soy sauce), mirin, lemon juice, sugar and sake combined in various quantities are used to make a myriad of delicious dishes. I substitute rice syrup or maple syrup for the sugar and now fancy myself as a regular Mrs Beeton of Tokyo. What's most exciting about lea rning to prepare some Japanese dishes is the introduction of seaweed to your cooking. After reading that seaweeds have the ability to prolong life, prevent disease and impart beauty and health, I was instantly hooked and made it my mission to find and create as many delicious dishes using the stuff as I could.

Dashi is to the Japanese what chicken stock is to the majority of westerners. It contains no fat and, as it's made with kombu, it is rich in minerals from the sea. Make a pot of dashi and delicious Japanese dishes are only minutes away.

10 cm (4 in) strip kombu
8 cups water
1 sachet dried bonito flakes − 5 g (⅙ oz)

makes 8 cups

Wipe each side of the kombu with a damp paper towel. Put the water and kombu in a large stockpot and heat over a medium heat until almost boiling. Remove and discard the kombu. Return the water to the heat and, to ensure it does not boil, add a further ¼ cup of cold water. Add the bonito flakes and, as soon as the water boils, remove the pot from the heat. Skim the surface of the water to remove the foam then, once the bonito flakes have sunk to the bottom, strain the liquid through a very fine sieve or a piece of gauze or muslin (cheesecloth).

Now that you've made the dashi, it's time to have some fun and create a range of sauces that can be used in some scrumptious dishes. Dashi can be stored in the fridge for up to 7 days or in the freezer for up to 3 months.

Use dashi in
- marinated watercress (page 30)
- tofu and soba miso soup (page 73)
- baked mushrooms and spinach with sesame sauce (page 116)
- Japanese eggplant (page 118)

dina's tomato sauce

Most working mothers throw together a quick dish of pasta and tomato sauce for the kids once a week. As a rule, I recommend that my clients stay away from pasta in the evenings, but there is no need to stay away from a great tomato sauce. The trick to a healthy pasta sauce that is rich in flavour and not bitter is to simmer it for at least 50 minutes. That way there's no need to use sugar. Not only is the sauce more flavoursome, it's much better for your health.

This recipe is from Dina, my friend John's cousin, who used to have an Italian restaurant in Adelaide. She came up to Sydney for a holiday and John set her to work in the kitchen, where she taught us to make all sorts of delicious, authentic Italian dishes. Taste the difference – it's all in the basil and using your hands to squash the tomatoes. For some reason, cutting the tomatoes with a knife makes the tomato sauce more acidic and bitter-tasting.

This sauce is a must for the toolkit, as it can be used as a base for so many different things. Of course the recipes in the list below will work with a bought sauce – just make sure you take select the one with the fewest additives.

3 tablespoons olive oil
1 cup fresh basil, chopped
1 medium-sized onion, finely chopped
3 cloves garlic, finely chopped
1 small carrot, peeled and finely chopped
1 chilli, seeded and finely sliced (optional)
4½ cups mixed fresh Italian herbs (thyme, oregano, parsley), chopped
4 x 400 g (14 oz) cans tomatoes

makes 4 cups

Heat the oil in a large saucepan until very hot, then drop in the basil and stir with a wooden spoon until it is crispy. Add the onion, garlic, carrot, chilli and Italian herbs and sauté until the vegetables are soft. Tip the tomatoes into a large bowl and break into small pieces with your hands. Add to the pan, bring to the boil and simmer for 45 minutes until the liquid has thickened and is reduced by almost half. Store the sauce in airtight containers in the fridge for up to 7 days, or freeze for up to 3 months.

Use Dina's tomato sauce in
- bean and tomato soup (page 70)
- Mediterranean fish stew (page 72)
- spinach and mushroom roll (page 106)
- clams and garlic polenta (page 146)

or as a base for homemade pizzas, vegetable tarts, with pasta or over baked fennel as an accompaniment to grilled meat or fish.

pastry

Making pastry is such a snack, particularly if you have a food processor. When you make your own pastry you can control the quantity of fat and flour you use. Try these basic pastry recipes and then experiment with different flours. Those with wheat allergies can make pastry from spelt flour. Remember that the pastry is just the canvas – it's what goes inside that makes it interesting. Roll the pastry as thin as you can and always remember to refrigerate it beforehand. A healthy flan served warm with salad makes a nice change from sandwiches at lunchtime.

I prefer using wholemeal flour for pastry. It has a higher fibre content and more nutrients are retained from milling the grain with the husk still intact. Wholemeal flour will make a heavier crust, so if you prefer to stick to white flour I urge you to buy unbleached. It may not look so pure but is undoubtedly better for you.

The wholemeal and oat pastry recipe is absolutely delicious in winter – it's heavy and hearty. It is packed full of fibre and will help lower your cholesterol with each mouthful (okay, that may be a slight exaggeration!). To make it, you'll need to use a non-hydrogenated table spread suitable for baking. Look in your local health food shop to find a suitable brand.

BASIC PASTRY

1¾ cups wholemeal plain (all-purpose) flour or spelt flour
½ teaspoon baking powder
pinch sea salt
¼ cup corn oil
½ cup cold water

makes 1 x 23 cm (8½ in) pastry shell or 48 mini tart shells

Preheat the oven to 180°C (350°F, Gas Mark 4). Mix the flour, baking powder and salt together put in a food processor. Mix in the corn oil using the dough attachment then slowly add the cold water until a dough forms. Put the dough in a plastic bag and chill for at least 30 minutes. Roll out the pastry evenly and line a lightly oiled 23 cm (8½ in) flan dish. Prick the pastry with a fork, cover with foil and weight with dried beans then bake in the centre of the oven for 15 minutes. Remove the weights and foil and bake the pastry for a further 5 minutes. Set aside to cool. The pastry is now ready to receive a delicious filling. If you're not using the pastry shell immediately, it will freeze for up to 3 months.

WHOLEMEAL AND OAT PASTRY

1 cup wholemeal plain (all-purpose) flour
¾ cup coarse oats
½ teaspoon baking powder
pinch sea salt
⅓ cup non-hydrogenated table spread
¼ cup cold water

makes 1 x 23 cm (8½ in) pastry shell or 48 mini tart shells

Follow the same method as above, adding the coarse oats to the flour and substituting the table spread for the corn oil.

Use pastry in
- tasty tartlets (page 59)
- balsamic onion, olive and tomato tart (page 110)
- vegetable and pesto tart (page 114)
- kumara, apple and onion tart (page 120)

beetroot

This root vegetable is so brightly coloured and so packed full of nutrients that it makes up part of my recipe toolkit. I often say to my clients, 'If it comes from the earth and it's a bright colour, then it is an anti-oxidant that can help fight disease and promote good health.' There's no vegetable brighter than the beetroot. (Don't be alarmed if your urine turns pink as a result of eating it!)

Most people throw out the beetroot leaves, but as they are also full of nutrient goodness it's worth having a recipe up your sleeve for them too. Beetroot greens (like silver beet or Swiss chard) contain oxalic acid, which can be harmful to the body. Steaming the leaves will remove toxins and leave you with a delicious, sweet-tasting salad leaf. The great news about beetroot is that, even with cooking, the nutrients remain intact. Pickling does reduce the level of nutrients but, as there are so many to start with, it is still a great healthy and delicious food.

ROAST BEETROOT
4 medium-sized beetroot (beet)
2 tablespoons olive oil
4 tablespoons water

Preheat the oven to 180°C (350°F, Gas Mark 4). Wash the beetroot and trim the top and bottom of the root without damaging the skin too much. Place on a baking tray with the oil and water. Tightly cover the baking tray with foil and bake for 45–60 minutes or until the beetroot is tender. Check after 25 minutes and baste with the liquid to ensure they don't dry out (add more water to the tray if required). Set aside to cool before peeling off the skin – wear gloves to protect your hands from staining.

PICKLED BEETROOT

2 cups good-quality white vinegar

¼ cup water

6 whole cloves

1 tablespoon allspice

2 x 500 ml (16 fl oz) jars

3 medium-sized roast beetroot (page 23)

makes 2 x 500 ml (16 fl oz) jars

Heat the vinegar and water with the cloves and allspice in a pan until close to boiling. Remove from the heat and leave to cool. Thoroughly wash two large glass jars with secure lids. To dry and sterilise the jars, place them on a baking tray in the oven on a very low heat (120°C, 250°F, Gas Mark 1) for 5–7 minutes. Cut each beetroot into eight even-sized pieces and place in the jars. Fill the jars with the cooled vinegar mix and leave for at least a week before eating. Store in the refrigerator.

BEETROOT GREENS

Thoroughly wash and trim the beetroot leaves, cutting the stalks about 5 cm (2 in) below the leaf. Place in a steamer and steam for 2 minutes. Remove from the heat and immediately refresh in cold water. Pat the leaves dry with a clean tea towel.

Use beetroot in

- fennel, beetroot leaf and olive salad with brazil nut pesto (page 86)
- beetroot, mango and goat's cheese salad (page 90)
- beetroot, orange and walnut salad (page 101)
- beetroot and sun-dried tomato salsa with blue-eye cod and green lentils (page 135)

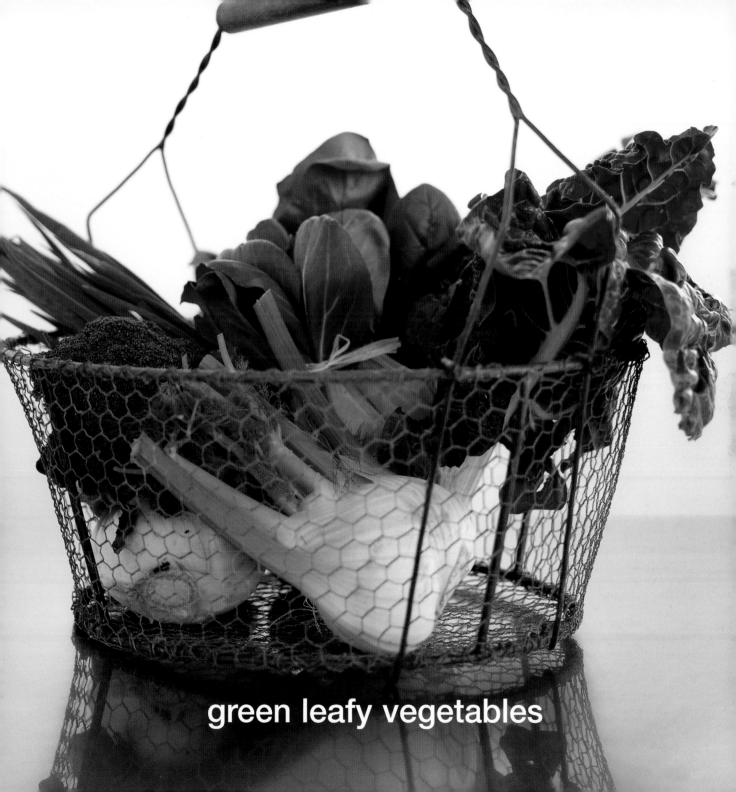

green leafy vegetables

asian salad

To make a salad for six, take four generous handfuls of any mix of three greens from those listed below. There is no hard and fast rule about which greens you choose, but it's nice if you are making an Asian salad to select leaves with an exotic-sounding name (even if they are grown at the back of Bourke). Tatsoi is a sweet little leaf and looks pretty mixed with the hardier looking mizuna. If you can't find these particular leaves, rocket (arugula), radicchio or any other mixed salad leaves will do (other than cos (romaine) and iceberg lettuce!).

greens
tatsoi
mizuna
mustard leaves
snow peas (mange-tout)

dressing
⅓ cup olive oil
1 tablespoon mirin
1 tablespoon brown rice vinegar
½ tablespoon tamari
1 small clove garlic, crushed

serves 6

Wash and dry the salad greens in a salad spinner. String the snow peas and arrange all the greens on a platter. To make the dressing, mix the ingredients in a jar. Pour over the greens and serve immediately. You can make up the dressing in advance and keep it in a jar in the fridge.

Serve Asian salad with
- sesame rice balls (page 64)
- lemon soy cutlets (page 109)
- kumara, apple and onion tart (page 120)
- calamari and lime salad (page 130)

italian green salad

You don't always have to make a big performance with greens (although they do often steal the show), but they must feature. Take a few handfuls of mixed leaves, top with shavings of fresh fennel (finocchio) and slices of avocado and dress with the best quality olive oil, a sprinkling of white wine vinegar and a little sea salt.

I hardly needed to write any of this – you've already got the recipe.

Serve Italian green salad with
- sun-dried tomato and sweetcorn omelette (page 62)
- Mediterranean fish stew (page 72)
- spinach and mushroom roll (page 106)
- redfish fishcakes with chilli jam (page 140)
- clams and garlic polenta (page 146)
- beefburgers with tomato and bean salsa (page 152)
- fillet steak with caper and olive salsa (page 158)

seasoned spinach and olive oil

Silver beet (Swiss chard) cooked badly is horrible. I'm sure those who think they don't like it were served it with the stalks left on. Silver beet stalks taste terrible. Grab the bunch, tear the leaves away from the stalks and throw the stalks away (or use them for compost). If you haven't enjoyed spinach in the past, have another go. Cooked properly it is delicious and works well with many recipes, particularly those listed below. I hope you like it – if you eat it regularly you'll soon be bursting out of your skin with health.

large bunch silver beet (Swiss chard)
pinch sea salt
1 tablespoon olive oil
za'tar, freshly ground black pepper, gomasio, dukka or lemon juice, to taste (optional)

serves 2–4 (depending on how much they love spinach)

Tear the leaves from the silver beet stalks and wash thoroughly in cold running water. Cut into smaller pieces along the veins of the leaf (see instructions for cutting vegetables 'energetically' on page 7). Add the salt to a large pan of water and bring to the boil. Add the silver beet, cover and cook for 2 minutes. Drain immediately and leave to cool slightly before squeezing out any excess moisture. Drizzle with olive oil and sprinkle with the za'tar, freshly ground black pepper, gomazio, dukka or lemon juice, or leave as is.

Serve seasoned spinach and olive oil with
- spicy black beans and pancakes with sweetcorn and caper salsa (page 76)
- grilled tuna and roast almond pesto (page 144)
- Moroccan lamb with fennel and olives (page 154)

stir-fried asian greens

It's late and you're tired. Open the fridge, pull out the greens and wash them. Heat the wok with a little sesame oil, throw in the veggies and 3 minutes later you're done. It is seriously that easy and seriously good for you.

1 tablespoon sesame oil
3 cloves garlic, finely sliced
6 spring onions (scallions), trimmed and cut into 5 cm (2 in) lengths
3 bunches bok choy, washed and trimmed
1 bunch broccolini, washed and trimmed
4 tablespoons tamari and mirin dressing or oyster sauce (see opposite)

serves 4

Heat the oil in a wok and stir-fry the garlic for 30 seconds. Add the spring onions, bok choy and broccolini and stir-fry until the vegetable stalks are cooked but still crisp. Remove from the wok and serve immediately with oyster sauce or tamari and mirin dressing (see opposite).

TAMARI AND MIRIN DRESSING

2 tablespoons tamari
2 tablespoons mirin

makes 4 tablespoons

Mix together the tamari and mirin and pour over the greens.

OYSTER SAUCE

Many supermarket brands of oyster sauce contain caramel, sugar and some preservatives. Check the label before buying, and make sure you get the one with the least additives and no preservatives. Better still, why not make your own?

1 x 500 ml (16 fl oz) jar fresh oysters (available from most good fish shops)
1 cup water
½ cup fish stock
½ teaspoon sea salt
1 clove garlic, crushed
1 spring onion (scallion), white portion only, finely chopped
1 small knob ginger, finely chopped
1 tablespoon cornflour (cornstarch) or crushed kudzu
1 tablespoon shoyu (soy sauce)
½ teaspoon maple syrup

makes 1 cup

Rinse the oyster meat in cold water. Place in a medium saucepan with the water, fish stock, sea salt, garlic, spring onion and ginger and bring to the boil over medium–high heat. Reduce the heat, partially cover and simmer for 30 minutes.

Mix the cornflour or kudzu with a little cold water to form a smooth paste. Add the shoyu and maple syrup, then gradually pour the mixture into the pan, stirring continuously. Simmer for another 10 minutes to allow the sauce to thicken, stirring occasionally to prevent sticking.

Pour the thickened sauce through a sieve into a sterilised jar with an airtight lid (discard the solid residue). Refrigerate once cool and keep in the fridge for up to 10 days.

Serving suggestions for stir-fried Asian greens
- savoury tofu (page 108)
- baked ocean trout with bean mash and Asian greens (page 124)
- blue-eye cod with papaya and beansprout salsa (serve the greens without sauce or dresssing) (page 126)
- baked Asian salmon (page 134)
- chicken kebabs (page 156)

marinated watercress

Liz Hurley recommends the watercress diet – apparently she lost a truckload of weight after childbirth by eating lashings of watercress soup. As Liz's career relies on her looking fabulous she has to endure some amount of physical hardship and sacrifice to restore her beauty and shape quickly! Most of us don't.

Many people today (Liz Hurley excluded) use watercress in much the same way they used to use parsley – as a decoration. It garnishes plates and is then thrown out. But I like it, and it is a good source of anti-oxidants. This dish is delicious and makes a fabulous accompaniment to grilled fish and sweetcorn.

2½ tablespoons dashi (page 19)
3 tablespoons mirin
4 tablespoons shoyu (soy sauce)
2 teaspoons pine nuts
4 bunches watercress

serves 4

Combine the dashi, mirin and shoyu in a pan over medium heat and bring to the boil. Remove from the heat and set aside to cool. Roast the pine nuts in a dry pan over medium heat until brown. Set aside to cool. Wash and trim the watercress, then boil in a large pan with plenty of lightly salted water for 2 minutes. Refresh in cold water and squeeze out any excess moisture. Cut into 2.5 cm (1 in) pieces, pour over the sauce and refrigerate for at least 30 minutes. Serve with roasted pine nuts on top.

tabouli

I'm trying to start a parsley revival, after being sworn off it for many years. As a child I used to find parsley the most unnecessary herb in the world: its sole purpose seemed to be to decorate plates of food at dinner parties. All soup arrived at the table with a blob of cream and a sprig of parsley on top and I was the one sent to the garden in the freezing cold to pick it. Now that I live in Australia I no longer associate parsley with freezing cold conditions and have promoted it back to its rightful place. Both tabouli and fatoush are delicious – they are wonderful as side salads, on their own or in sandwiches.

½ cup burghul (bulgur)
8–10 spring onions (scallions)
2 teaspoons salt
¼ teaspoon freshly ground black pepper
¼ teaspoon mixed spice or nutmeg
5 cups finely chopped fresh flat-leaf parsley
¼ cup fresh mint, finely chopped
3 large tomatoes, diced
¼ cup lemon juice
¼ cup olive oil

serves 6

To prepare the burghul, wash and rinse, then squeeze any excess moisture from it before refrigerating for at least 1 hour. Trim and finely chop the spring onions. Add to the burghul with the salt, pepper and spice. Add the parsley, mint and tomatoes and refrigerate until ready to serve. Just before serving, add the lemon juice and oil and toss well.

fatoush

A variation on tabouli, fatoush is another dish from the Middle East. I particularly enjoy it with fish. The capers, rocket and sesame seeds give it quite an unusual flavour. Traditional fatoush has flatbread broken through it, but this version is a marvellous alternative for anyone with a wheat allergy. I promised my yoga teacher, Nicole, who gave me this recipe, I would mention that her mother and sister invented it.

1 tablespoon sesame seeds
1 large bunch flat-leaf parsley
½ bunch mint
1 bunch baby rocket (arugula)
6 spring onions (scallions), chopped
3 vine-ripened tomatoes
2 Lebanese cucumbers
3 tablespoons capers
juice of 2 lemons
pinch sea salt

serves 4

Dry-roast the sesame seeds in a pan until they turn slightly golden. Set aside to cool. Wash and dry the parsley, mint and rocket. Using a sharp knife, chop the herbs finely (a blunt knife will bruise the leaves), then finely chop the spring onions, tomatoes and cucumbers. Rinse the capers and chop finely. Mix with the herbs and vegetables, pour over the lemon juice and sprinkle with the sea salt and sesame seeds.

If you are serving the salad with fish, put the fish on a platter with the fatoush around it and kumara chips (see page 66) on top.

green bean, pine nut and garlic salad with raspberry vinaigrette

This lovely salad is from Karla Maverick, my macrobiotic cooking teacher. Karla served it with pinto beans and miso dressing, pickles, seaweed and brown rice – all very delicious. You can elect to go down the macrobiotic road with this salad or simply serve it with a piece of grilled fish or chicken. It's delicious either way.

2 cloves garlic
¼ cup pine nuts
3 handfuls green beans

vinaigrette
1 tablespoon raspberry vinegar
1 teaspoon wholegrain mustard
½ teaspoon dry mustard
1 teaspoon rice syrup
pinch sea salt
¼ cup olive oil
1 clove garlic, bruised

serves 6

Using a small fine knife or vegetable peeler, cut thin slivers of garlic and put them on a piece of paper towel to blot dry. Dry-roast the pine nuts in a heavy-based frying pan. Add the garlic and toss the nuts and garlic slivers regularly until they become golden. Wash then top and tail the green beans, then steam them for 3–5 minutes until they are bright green and still crunchy. Remove from the heat and plunge into cold water to help retain their colour and stop further cooking.

To make the vinaigrette, whisk the vinegar, mustards, rice syrup and salt together until well blended. Gradually add the oil and finally the whole garlic clove. Allow the dressing to stand and the garlic to infuse for at least 20 minutes before serving.

Toss the dressing through the beans and serve with the garlic and pine nuts sprinkled on top.

I remember seeing a motivational speaker years ago who spoke about the four critical factors for good life and good health – they were breakfast, fish, laughter and sex! I can't help you with the other three, but hopefully you'll take some of these breakfast recipes on board and be 25 per cent of the way towards health and happiness. If you've got the sex part sewn up, you'll be in need of a good breakfast anyway!

Ask those you consider to be healthy what their favourite meal of the day is and I bet that they'll say breakfast. It is the most important meal of the day. A good breakfast will boost the metabolism, kick-start your day, accelerate the removal of food 'residue' from your system, and provide enough energy for body and mind to function efficiently for most of the morning. We are all aware of the role fibre plays in the diet, but few are aware of how hard it can be to consume the recommended daily intake of fibre (which is 30 g or 1 oz). A breakfast of whole grains, fruit and nuts would have to be the easiest way to consume a large percentage of this recommended daily intake.

breakfasts

bircher muesli

" There are hundreds of Bircher muesli recipes out there, but many are made with cream or full-fat yoghurt. This version is simple and tastes delicious. Served with a few blueberries, it also looks beautiful. Berries are **packed full of anti-oxidants,** so when they are in season eat lots of them – although I once used frozen berries at a function when berries were out of season and, between you and me, they were lovely. Bircher muesli is definitely worth getting up for and is best served the day after making. **""**

1½ cups oats

¼ cup almond slivers

¼ cup pear juice concentrate

juice of ½ lemon

1 cup grated apple or pear

1 cup low-fat natural yoghurt

serves 4

Mix the oats and almonds in a bowl and stir through the pear juice concentrate, lemon juice and grated fruit. Gradually mix in the yoghurt until the mixture is quite sloppy. Cover and leave overnight. Add more yoghurt in the morning if the mixture is too thick.

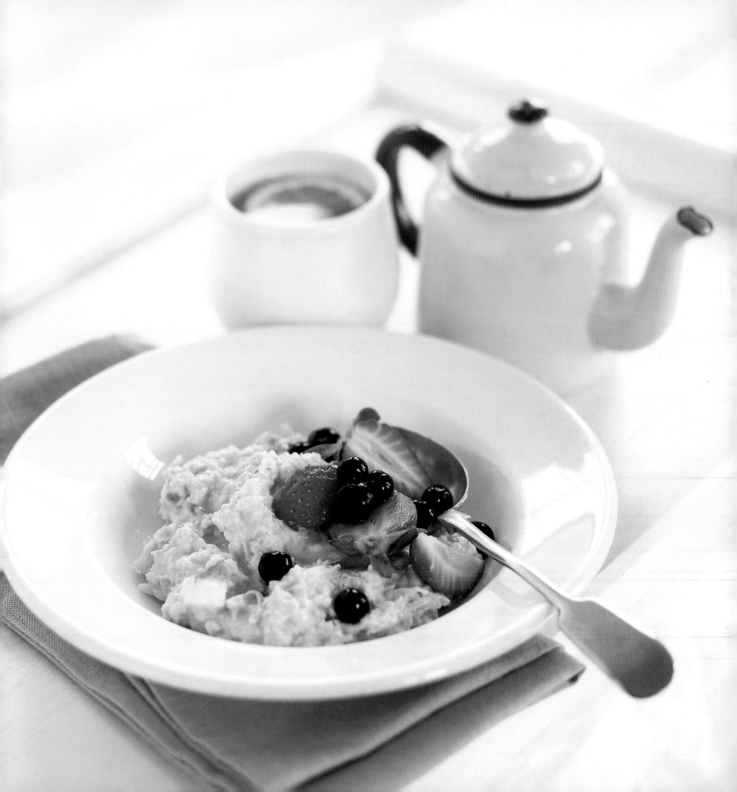

a cleansing start

"Don't ever get the idea that skipping breakfast is okay. It's not, especially if you are trying to lose weight by cutting out bread, pasta and rice at night. Your body needs food for fuel and energy at the start of the day. It will help start the digestive process, boost the metabolism and sustain energy for the morning. This very quick and simple high-fibre cereal is a favourite with most of my clients, who generally agree that it keeps them fuelled for the whole morning with no pangs of hunger at all."

1 cup rolled oats

½ cup LSA (ground linseeds, sunflower seeds and almonds – available from health food shops)

½ cup barley flakes

½ cup rye flakes

½ cup dried prunes, chopped

makes about 14 serves

Mix all the ingredients together and store in an airtight container in the fridge. Use about 4 dessertspoons per serve and add fresh fruit and natural yoghurt. For an added cleansing effect, put 1 tablespoon of flaxseed (linseed) oil on top.

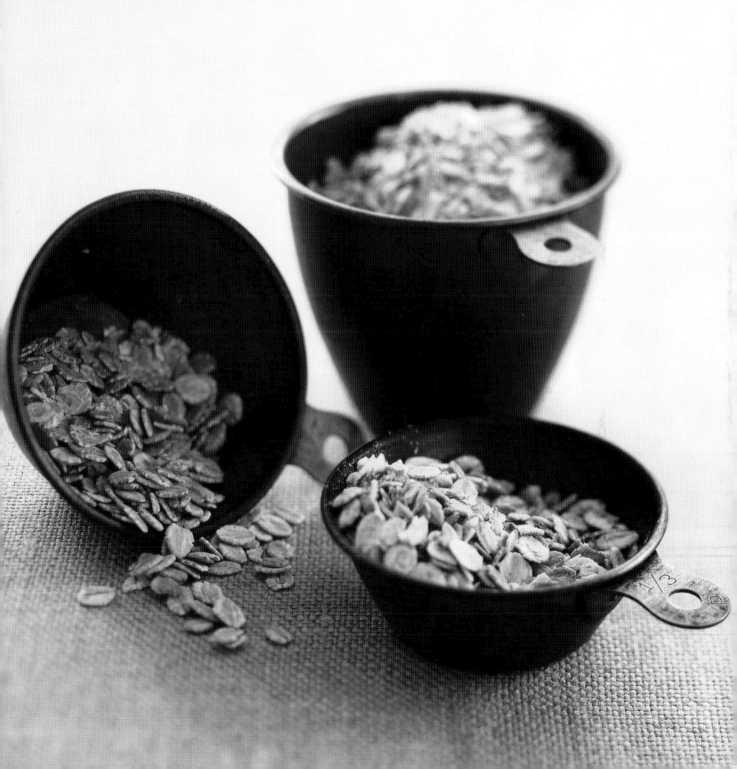

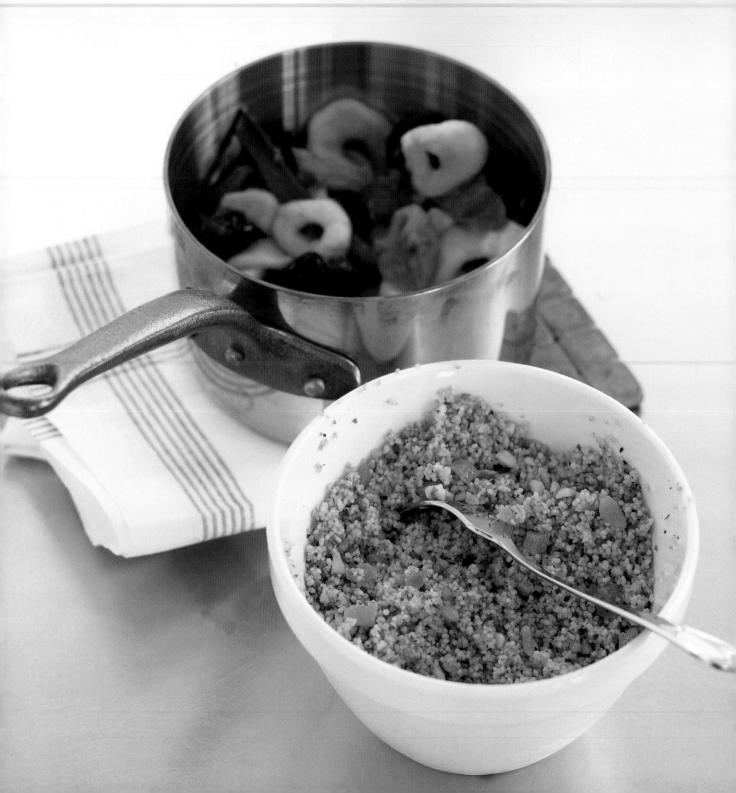

breakfast couscous

" Couscous is crushed semolina and is usually eaten with savoury foods. It is a good source of protein and provides a **great energising start** to the day. This breakfast recipe is tasty and delicious, especially in winter, served with stewed fruit and yoghurt. **""**

1 cup couscous

½ cup mixed chopped nuts (almonds, brazil nuts, walnuts)

1½ cups water

½ cup apple juice concentrate

¼ cup dried apricots, chopped

fresh fruit or stewed fruit compote (see over), to serve

low-fat natural yoghurt, to serve

serves 4

Roast the couscous in a dry frying pan for a minute or two until the grain darkens very slightly and gives off a fragrant, toasty aroma. Set aside in a glass bowl. Roast the nuts in the same way, taking care not to burn them, and set aside. In a small pan, bring the water and apple concentrate to a boil. Pour the liquid into the bowl of couscous, cover with plastic wrap and set aside for 5 minutes. Remove the plastic and, using a fork, separate the couscous grains. Stir through the nuts and apricots and serve with fresh or stewed fruit and yoghurt. Breakfast couscous keeps fresh for up to 3 days in the fridge.

stewed fruit compote

" One of my testers said that the smell of this dish reminded her of Christmas. How delightful to be mentally transported to a happy holiday every time you open the fridge! Food should always **make you happy** (and healthy). This recipe is very high in fibre and makes a delicious accompaniment to winter porridge, or yoghurt. **""**

1 cup dried apricots

1 cup dried apples

1 cup dried pitted prunes

½ cup dried figs

2 cinnamon sticks (or large piece of cassia bark)

zest of 1 lemon

juice of 1 lemon

Put the dried fruits in a saucepan and pour over enough water to cover them. Add the cinnamon sticks, lemon zest and lemon juice and slowly bring the mixture to a boil, then simmer over a low heat for 50 minutes or until the fruit is tender but not falling apart. Allow to cool, remove the cinnamon sticks or cassia bark and serve. The compote will keep in the fridge for up to 5 days.

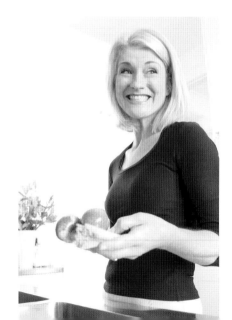

mixed grain porridge

" This will put hairs on your chest. I never knew what that meant, but I do know that this will fuel you for the whole morning with **energy to spare**. I have certainly eaten enough bowls of porridge to know that the energy part is true, and I am pleased to tell you that, despite all the bowls of porridge I've consumed in my life, I don't have any hairs on my chest! This recipe does take quite a long time, so you might prefer to save it for a weekend when you want a leisurely start to the day, or to make it in a slow cooker (crockpot) overnight, ready for breakfast the next day. "

1 cup coarse oatmeal

½ cup barley

6 cups water

2 cups apple juice

1 teaspoon sea salt

1 tablespoon grated ginger

½ cup slivered almonds, dry-roasted
   (optional)

¼ cup chopped dried apricots

fresh fruit or stewed fruit compote
   (page 42), to serve

serves 4

Rinse the oatmeal and barley, pour over enough cold water to cover and leave to soak overnight. The next morning, drain the grains and put in a pan with the water, apple juice and sea salt. Bring the porridge to the boil, stirring continuously, then reduce the heat and simmer for 35–40 minutes. Stir the porridge regularly to ensure it doesn't stick to the bottom of the pan. Once the majority of the liquid has been absorbed into the grain, add the ginger, almonds and apricots and continue to cook for a further 15 minutes or until the porridge reaches a fairly thick consistency. Serve with fresh or stewed fruit.

buckwheat pancakes with rhubarb, yoghurt and ginger

" Rhubarb and parsley are about the only things that I can remember growing in our garden when I was a child. I'm certain it wasn't because my parents were overly health-conscious, but both are **excellent sources of calcium**. For those of you who are lactose intolerant, it is useful to know that the lactose is broken down in buttermilk and yoghurt. Many people also find sheep and goat's yoghurt easier to digest. I really like the taste of sheep's yoghurt and I love this recipe – it's healthy and looks splendid. "

sheep's yoghurt, to serve

rhubarb

1 bunch rhubarb

2 tablespoons pear concentrate

1 tablespoon grated ginger

3 tablespoons water

pancakes

1 cup buckwheat flour

¼ teaspoon salt

¼ teaspoon baking powder

1 large egg

2 cups buttermilk (or 1½ cups soy milk if non-dairy is preferred)

1 tablespoon corn oil

makes 6 pancakes

To make the topping, trim and wash the rhubarb stalks then cut into 2.5 cm (1 in) pieces. Place the rhubarb, pear concentrate, ginger and water in a heavy-based pan, cover with a tight-fitting lid and place over a low to medium heat. Test the rhubarb after 5 minutes and continue to check every 2 minutes thereafter until it is soft and tender. Set aside to cool slightly while you make the pancakes. The rhubarb will keep in a covered container in the fridge for up to 4 days.

To make the pancakes, sift the buckwheat flour, salt and baking powder into a bowl. Make a well in the centre. Beat the egg and buttermilk together in a separate bowl, then pour into the well and whisk into the dry ingredients until bubbles appear on the surface and the batter is smooth and runny. Pour the pancake mixture into a jug, cover with plastic wrap and set aside for 20 minutes.

Grease a small pancake pan with the oil and wipe off the excess with paper towel. Place the pan over a medium heat and, when hot, pour in sufficient mixture to make a pancake about 2 mm (¹⁄₁₆ in) thick. The pancake is ready to turn once you see little air holes appearing on the uncooked surface. Flip the pancake and cook until golden, then repeat the process until the batter mixture is finished. Stack the cooked pancakes on a plate and keep warm in a slow oven (150°C, 300°F, Gas Mark 2) as you cook the rest. To serve, spoon the rhubarb topping over the pancakes and top with sheep's yoghurt.

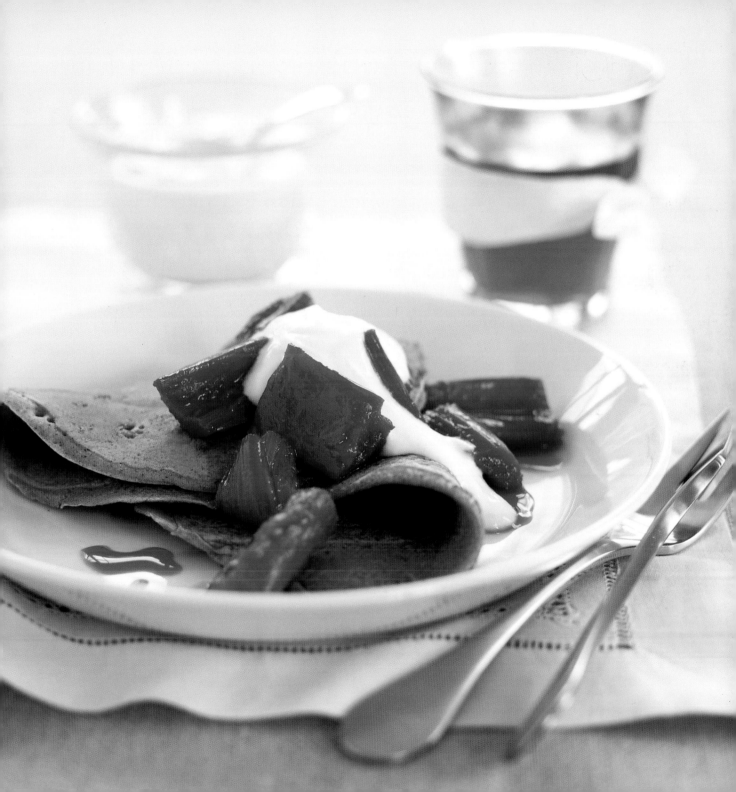

poached pears with fromage blanc, oats and honey

" Many chefs will rear up in horror at the idea of leaving the skin on pears, but the skin is high in fibre, so I recommend that you leave it on. This is a particularly **lovely dish in winter**. Fromage blanc is very mild, soft cheese with a whipped texture not dissimilar to thick cream. If you can't find fromage blanc, use cottage cheese or ricotta. "

4 pears

3 cups water

1 cup pear juice concentrate

1 tablespoon grated ginger

juice of ½ lemon

½ cup rolled oats

¼ cup walnuts

3 tablespoons honey

125 g (4 oz) fromage blanc

serves 4

Cut the pears into quarters, removing the core from each quarter. Bring the water, pear juice concentrate, ginger and lemon juice to a simmer in a large pan. Drop in the pear quarters, cover the pan and simmer very slowly until the pears are tender (the time will vary, so allow 20–45 minutes to be safe). Meanwhile, dry-roast the oats and walnuts in a frying pan over a moderate heat and warm the honey in a small pan. Serve the pears with the oat and walnut mixture on top, add a spoonful of fromage blanc and drizzle over the warmed honey.

crunchy nut muesli

" With this in the cupboard, there's no excuse for skipping breakfast. There are hundreds of delicious organic muesli products you can buy, but it's **lots of fun to make your own** – and better for you. This recipe makes about 500 g (1 lb), but you can easily reduce the quantities. Nuts are high in omega-3 fats and are very good for you. Once chopped, heated and exposed to air and light, however, they can become rancid and lose much of their nutritional goodness. The best advice is to buy the nuts whole, store them in a cool, dry place and, once cooked and chopped, eat within a week. This muesli is delicious, so that shouldn't be too hard a task! "

1 cup rolled oats

½ cup rye flakes

½ cup barley flakes

½ cup roughly chopped macadamia
   nuts

½ cup roughly chopped almonds

½ cup roughly chopped brazil nuts

½ cup chopped dried apple

½ cup chopped dried apricots

¼ cup maple syrup

milk or soy milk, to serve

makes 500 g (1 lb)

Preheat the oven to 180°C (350°F, Gas Mark 4). Mix all the cereals, nuts and dried fruit together in a bowl. Gently heat the maple syrup in a small pan until it becomes very runny then pour over the mixture and toss to coat. Spread the coated mixture on a non-stick baking sheet and roast in the oven for 20 minutes, tossing frequently. Cool and store in an airtight container for up to a week. Serve with your milk of preference.

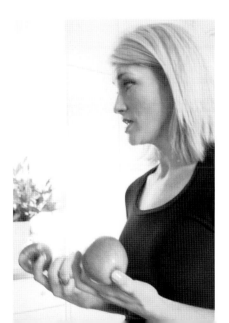

In my opinion, entertaining should be easy. A typical dinner party at my place starts with guests grazing on tasty little bits of food that can be prepared well in advance. A big platter in the middle of the table seems to help get things off to an easy start, as your guests get to know each other while they pass the food around.

Sweep the platter away and serve a delicious (and light) main course followed by an even lighter dessert. Your guests will never suspect that you've subjected them to an evening of 'food coaching', but will leave the table feeling sated and ready for a restful night's sleep. The recipes in this section can be mixed and matched, served at dinner or lunch or even at a casual evening drinks party.

dips, snacks & finger food

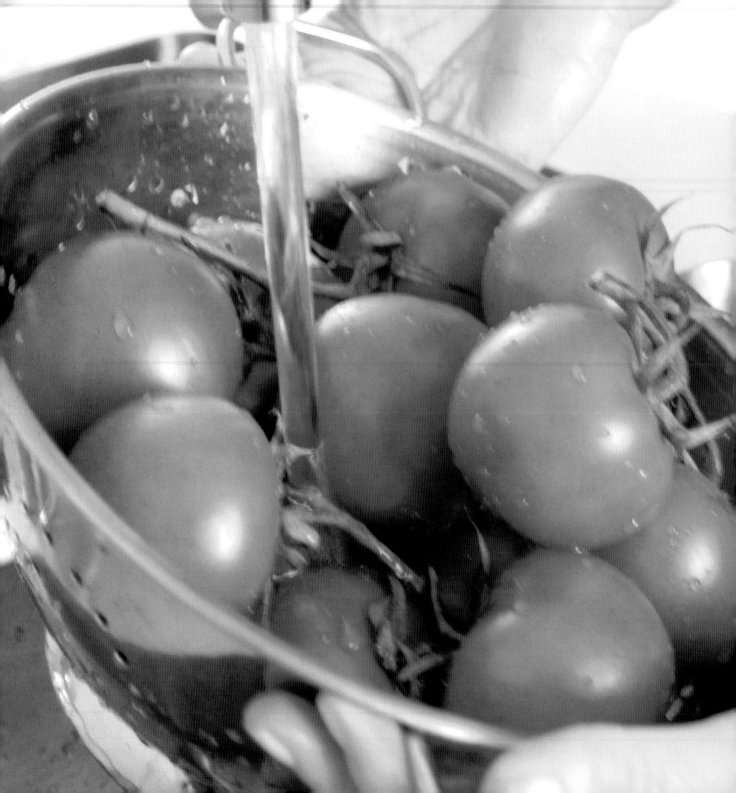

middle eastern mezze

"Your **guests will enjoy** picking their way through this lovely mezze. None of the components is hard to prepare and most can be done hours in advance. Before you start this dish, make sure you have a pastry brush. I am all for the cholesterol-lowering properties of olive oil, but I don't think we need to eat our food swimming in it. Fill a little bowl with oil and use a pastry brush to lightly coat the vegetables, bread and fish. This is much better than using those horrible sprays, which invariably miss the food and end up all over the kitchen."

crispy middle eastern bread

6 slices flat bread

olive oil for brushing

1 tablespoon nigella seeds

2 tablespoons za'tar (page 15)

Preheat the oven to 180°C (350°F, Gas Mark 4). Tear the bread into pieces – the more irregular the better. Brush the pieces with olive oil and lightly sprinkle half of them with nigella seeds and the other half with za'tar. Heat the bread in the oven for 7–10 minutes until golden brown. Leave to cool.

roast tomatoes

9 Roma (plum) tomatoes

1 tablespoon olive oil

1 teaspoon chilli oil >

Preheat the oven to 120°C (250°F, Gas Mark 1). Slice the tomatoes in half. Mix together the olive oil and chilli oil and brush over each tomato half. Roast for 3 hours. >

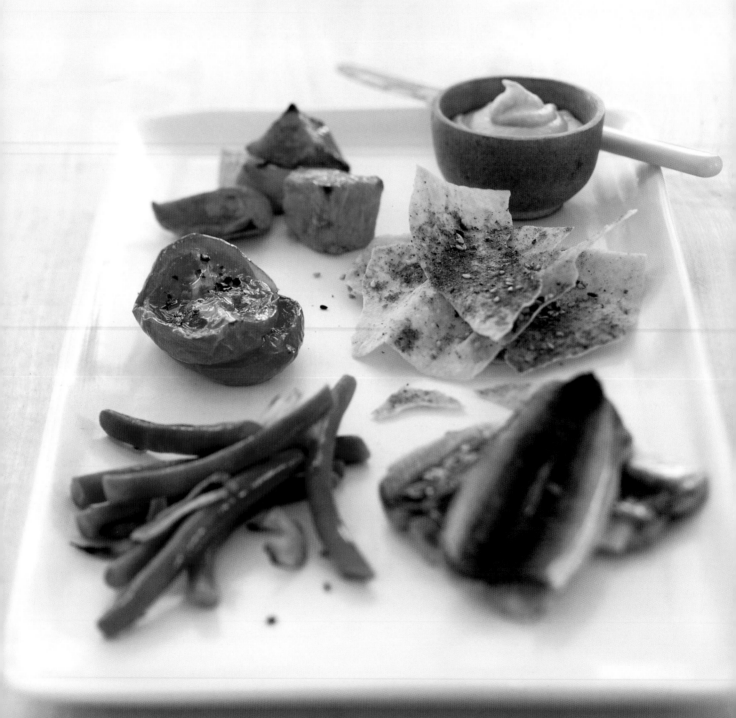

mezze continued

grilled sardines

200 g (6½ oz) fresh sardine fillets

juice of 1 lemon

olive oil for brushing

sea salt, to taste

freshly ground black pepper, to taste

Wipe the fillets with a clean, damp cloth and pat dry. With a knife, gently score the skin of each fillet twice, about 2.5 cm (1 in) apart. Squeeze the lemon juice over the fillets and brush each one with olive oil. Season to taste. Preheat a char-grill pan or barbecue and grill the fillets, skin-side down, for 2 minutes or until the skin is crispy. The sardines will cook through in this time without turning.

roast kumara

1 medium-sized kumara (sweet potato)

olive oil for brushing

Preheat the oven to 180°C (350°F, Gas Mark 4). Peel and slice the kumara into pieces about 2.5 cm (1 in) thick. Blot off any moisture with dry paper towel and brush each piece with olive oil. Bake for 25 minutes, turning occasionally.

steamed beans with crunchy garlic shavings

5 cloves garlic, thinly sliced

400 g (13 oz) green beans

juice of ½ lemon

1 tablespoon olive oil

1 quantity hummus (page 18)

serves 6

Preheat the oven to 180°C (350°F, Gas Mark 4). Roast the garlic slices for 10 minutes, turning occasionally. (If you are cooking all the mezze together, you can put the garlic into the oven to one side of the kumara 10 minutes before the end of the cooking time.) Top and tail the beans and steam for 6 minutes. Remove from the heat, drizzle with the lemon juice and olive oil and sprinkle the garlic shavings over the top.

white bean and dill dip

" This dip, like hummus, can be used in many ways. It's lower in fat than hummus, but still high in fibre, so it's **good news all round** for those wishing to lose weight. Grab the food processor, a cup of beans, some garlic, dill and olive oil and it's done – literally in minutes. If you are going to use canned beans, try to buy organic ones. "

1 cup canned or cooked (see
    page 177–8) haricot (navy) or
    cannellini beans

2 cloves garlic, crushed

1 tablespoon olive oil

2 tablespoons chopped fresh dill

2 tablespoons miso dressing
    (page 15)

makes about 1 cup

Drain the beans and put in the food processor with the garlic, olive oil and dill. Blend, slowly adding the miso dressing until the mixture develops a creamy dip consistency. Serve with raw vegetables or crispy Middle Eastern bread (page 51).

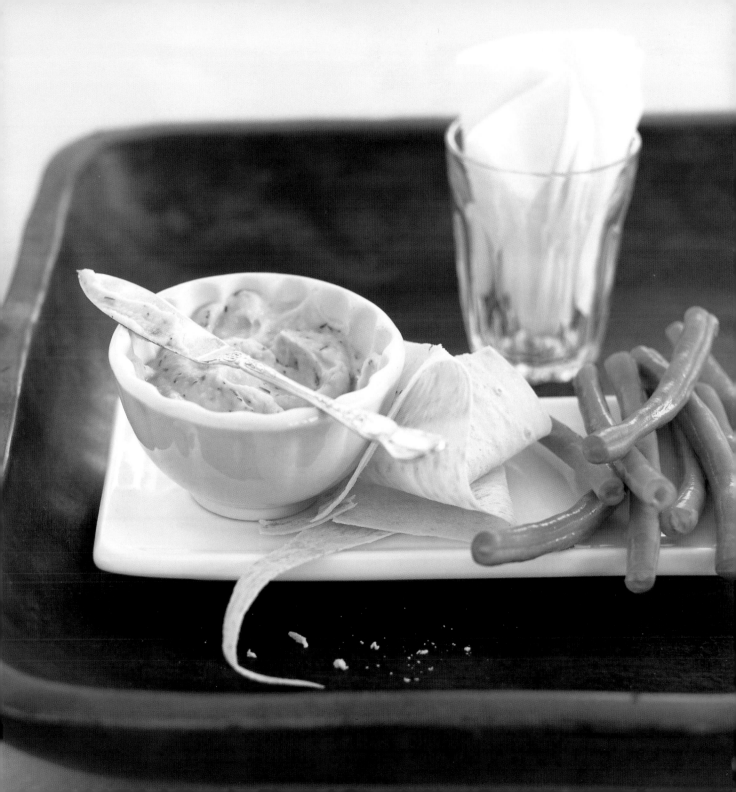

scottish oatcakes

" I used to love my mother's oatcakes. Served with honey and cheddar cheese they were the perfect after-school snack. Traditional oatcakes were made using lard (or in more affluent households, butter). It's a shame to negate the **cholesterol-lowering properties** of oats by using butter, so I've replaced it with a table spread, available at health food shops, that contains no hydrogenated, hardened or trans fatty acids – all of which have been linked with heart disease – no dairy and no cholesterol. **"**

1⅓ cups coarse oatmeal

½ cup wholemeal self-raising
(self-rising) flour

pinch sea salt

½ cup non-hydrogenated table spread

2 tablespoons chilled water

makes 35–40 oatcakes

Using the dough blade of your food processor, mix together the oats, flour, salt and spread. Process until the mixture resembles coarse breadcrumbs then slowly add chilled water until the mixture forms a stiff dough. Stop at this point, even if you haven't used all the water. Place the dough in a plastic bag and put in the freezer for about 20 minutes (or as long as it takes you to clean up the mess and drink a glass of water). Preheat the oven to 180°C (350°F, Gas Mark 4). Remove the dough from the plastic bag and roll it out on a floured board to about 3 mm (⅛ in) thickness. Cut into rounds about 5 cm (2 in) in diameter, place on a non-stick baking sheet and bake for 15–20 minutes or until golden.

Serve Scottish oatcakes with

- stewed strawberries and goat's curd
- honey (perfect for kids)
- beetroot, orange and walnut salad (page 101)
- poached dried figs (page 170)

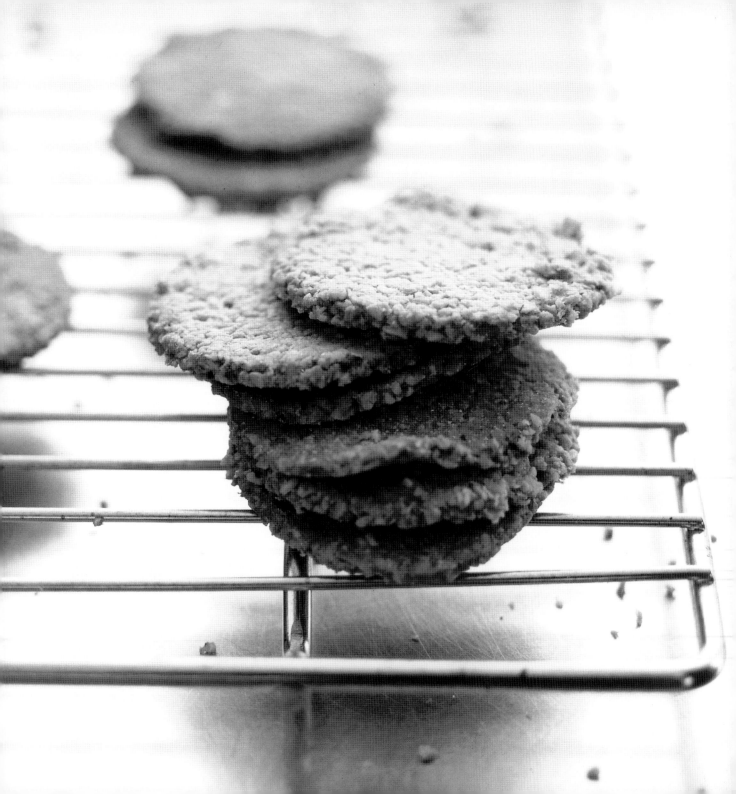

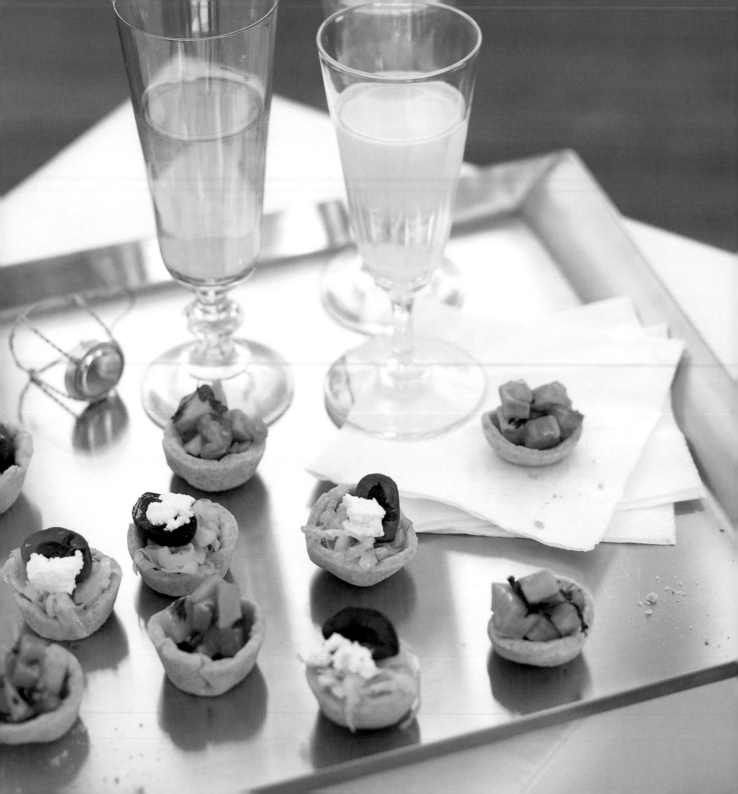

tasty tartlets

"Typical party food is almost certainly going to assault your body. Creamy dips, cheeses and spring rolls (the deep-fried ones) are just some of the horrors that spring to mind. Not only is the food unhealthy (and horrible), it can be quite expensive. These little tarts are easy and inexpensive. The pastry shells can be made in advance and frozen. Defrost them on the day and you can make the fillings in less than an hour."

1 quantity basic pastry (page 21)

kumara filling

½ large kumara (sweet potato), peeled
   and cut into 5 mm (¼ in) cubes

5 vine-ripened tomatoes, cut into
   small cubes

1 cup chopped fresh chervil

sea salt, to taste

leek filling

1 tablespoon corn oil

2 leeks, washed and sliced

¼ cup pitted kalamata olives, cut
   into quarters

2 tablespoons soft goat's cheese
   (chèvre)

makes 48 tartlets (24 of each filling)

Make your pastry following the toolkit recipe instructions, using a mini-muffin tin and reducing the cooking time to 10 minutes with the weights on and 5 minutes with them removed.

For the kumara filling, preheat the oven to 160°C (325°F, Gas Mark 3). Place the kumara and tomatoes in a lightly oiled roasting tin and sprinkle with the chervil. Season with sea salt and roast for 35 minutes. Fill half the pastry cases with the mixture.

For the leek filling, heat the oil in a large, heavy-based saucepan and sauté the leeks over a low heat for 15 minutes. They will reduce considerably in volume and become very soft and sweet. Let them cool, then put a little in each of the remaining pastry cases, topping with a couple of olive quarters and a small amount of goat's cheese.

Gently heat the tartlets in a 150°C (300°F, Gas Mark 2) oven for a few minutes before serving.

fresh spring rolls

"These are real spring rolls, **fresh and clean-tasting**. Their flavour is derived from the fresh vegetables and herbs and not overwhelmed by a thick, greasy batter. If you don't have time to wrap the rolls up yourself you can either mix all the ingredients together and serve them in individual bowls or put a large bowl on the table with the rice paper and your guests can wrap up their own. **"**

1 cup rice vermicelli noodles

1 teaspoon sesame oil

1 large clove garlic, crushed

1 red chilli, seeded and finely
   chopped

1 tablespoon rice syrup

juice of 1 lime

1 large carrot, peeled and grated

1 cup beansprouts, cut into 1 cm
   (½ in) pieces

½ cup chopped fresh coriander
   (cilantro)

½ cup chopped fresh mint

½ cup chopped organic peanuts

cracked black pepper, to taste

rice paper (larger, square sheets are
   best)

dipping sauce

3 tablespoons shoyu (soy sauce)

3 tablespoons mirin

1 teaspoon sesame seeds

makes 6 large rolls

Soak the vermicelli noodles in a bowl of boiling water for 5 minutes or until soft. Meanwhile, heat the sesame oil in a small saucepan and sauté the garlic and chilli for 2 minutes. Add the rice syrup and lime juice to the pan and stir well. Drain the noodles and rinse in cold water to remove any sticky starch. Cut the noodles into pieces about 2.5 cm (1 in) long to ease the rolling process. Mix the garlic and chilli through the noodles, then add the other vegetables, herbs and nuts. Combine well and season with pepper.

To make the rolls, dip a sheet of rice paper into hot water. Lay the softened rice paper on the workbench and spoon a small amount of noodle salad about a third of the way from the front of the sheet, leaving room at the sides to fold the paper in. Make sure you don't overfill the rolls or it will be difficult to roll them. Lift the front of the sheet over the mixture, tuck the sides in and then tightly roll the remaining paper around the parcel. Practice makes perfect and, even if your first attempts don't look too beautiful, they will still taste delicious!

To make the dipping sauce, mix the shoyu and mirin together in a bowl and sprinkle the sesame seeds on top.

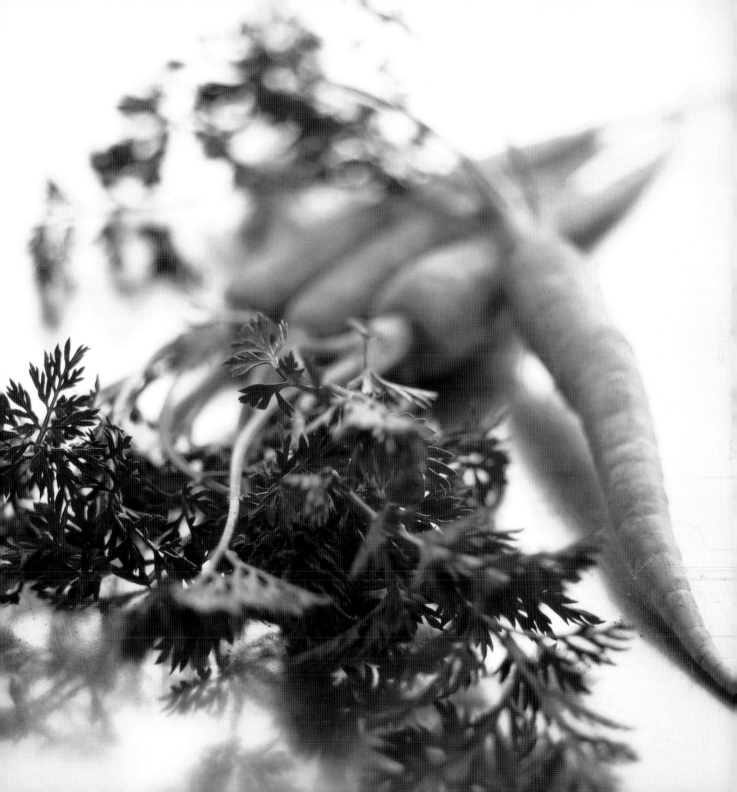

sun-dried tomato and sweetcorn omelette

" 'Ho hum', you may cry, but an omelette is not so ho hum when you use the delicious contrasting flavours of sweetcorn and slightly tangy sun-dried tomatoes. Serve this up with salad and you have a very quick, delicious, healthy meal. "

1 cob (ear) corn

4 eggs

½ cup skim milk

sea salt, to taste

cracked black pepper, to taste

1 teaspoon olive oil

10 sun-dried tomatoes, drained and
    chopped into small pieces

2 servings Italian green salad
    (page 27)

serves 2

Steam the corn cob for 3–5 minutes. Remove the cob from the pan and set aside. Beat the eggs with the skimmed milk and season with salt and pepper. Using a clean tea towel to hold the corn cob, cut off the corn kernels and reserve in a bowl. Heat the olive oil over medium heat in a small non-stick omelette pan and coat the bottom of the pan. Add half the egg mixture and roll it around the pan until the bottom is covered and the bottom layer begins to cook (lift the cooked mixture off the edges of the pan to prevent it from sticking). When the mixture is firm underneath but still runny on top, drop in half the tomatoes and half the corn. Place the pan under the grill (broiler) until the egg is cooked and the corn is slightly toasted and crunchy. Repeat the process to create the second omelette and serve with the Italian green salad.

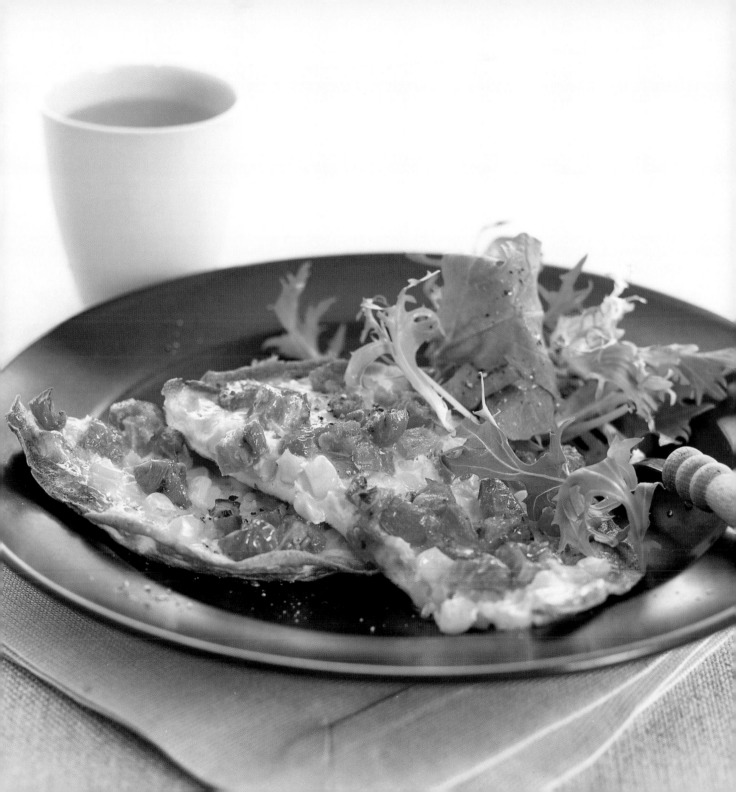

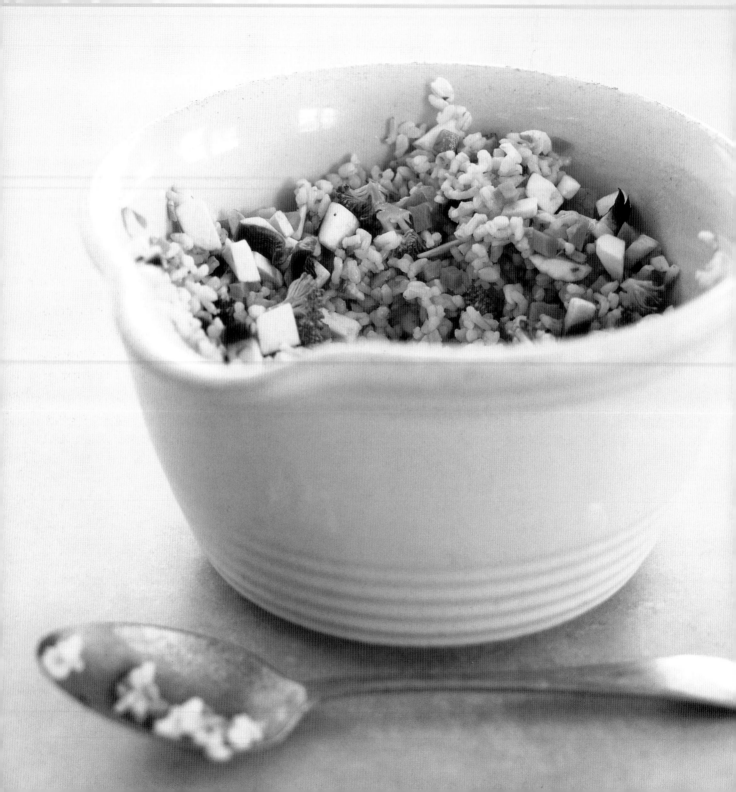

sesame rice balls

"Now that it is the thing to eat whole grains – and other foods our ancestors ate – it's time to make leftovers fashionable. But that's not to say we should go down the road of bubble and squeak, where everything is thrown together and fried! These rice balls could have guests fooled into thinking you've been slaving over a hot stove for hours. They are delicious and make an ideal lunch (or make them smaller and serve as finger food at a party)."

1 cup mixed raw vegetables (broccoli, carrots, zucchinis and mushrooms)

3 cups cold cooked short-grain brown rice

2 tablespoons tahini

juice of ½ lemon

1 tablespoon tamari

½ cup silken tofu

1 cup sesame seeds

Asian salad (page 26), to serve

dipping sauce

2 tablespoons tamari

2 tablespoons mirin

makes 18 rice balls

Chop the vegetables very finely – if the vegetable pieces are too big, the mixture will not stick together. Combine the rice and vegetables in a bowl. Mix the tahini, lemon juice, tamari and tofu in a blender until smooth and creamy. Pour this sauce over the rice and vegetables and mix thoroughly. Preheat the oven to 180°C (350°F, Gas Mark 4). With wet hands, roll bits of the rice mixture into balls of about 5 cm (2 in) diameter. Roll the balls in the sesame seeds until they are completely coated and place them on a baking tray. Bake for 40 minutes, turning the balls twice during the baking process.

While the balls are cooking, make the dipping sauce by mixing the tamari and mirin together in a small bowl. Serve the rice balls with Asian salad and a separate dish of dipping sauce on the side.

moroccan couscous

" Couscous is a delicious substitute for rice and takes so much less time to prepare. Many **people with wheat allergies** find that they can still eat wheat if it is unbaked. So, while bread is a problem, noodles and couscous can be tolerated. Certain schools of thought suggest that wheat intolerance develops from eating too much refined flour – in breads, cakes and biscuits (cookies), but the grain in couscous is still pretty much intact when it is ground. Buy the organic wholegrain couscous – it tastes much better.

This dish is *so* good served with simple baked fish and some greens. Come home from work, whack the fish in foil and bake in the oven and, while that's cooking, make up the couscous. With steamed greens it looks (and tastes) delicious. **" "**

½ cup slivered almonds

2 cups couscous

1 tablespoon olive oil

2 cloves garlic, crushed

2 red chillies, seeded and finely chopped

2 cups boiling water

1 x 4 cm (1½ in) piece preserved lemon, cut into thin slivers (page 16)

1 cup chopped fresh parsley

1 tablespoon nigella seeds

kumara chips (optional)

1 medium-sized kumara (sweet potato)

serves 4

To make the kumara chips, preheat the oven to 150°C (300°F, Gas Mark 2). Using a vegetable peeler, peel off and discard the skin, then peel thin slices (chips) off the kumara. Lay the chips on a flat, very lightly greased, baking sheet in a single layer. Bake for about 15 minutes, then turn the chips over. Keep moving them around on the tray every few minutes until they have all dried out and become crisp. Remove from the oven and leave to cool.

Preheat the oven to 180°C (350°F, Gas Mark 4). Roast the almonds on a baking sheet for 4 minutes or until they turn golden (keep your eye on them, as they can burn very quickly). In a dry pan roast the couscous until it produces a lovely aroma, then put aside. Heat the oil in the same pan and sauté the garlic and chilli until soft. Return the grain to the pan then stir through the garlic and chilli. Remove from the heat, add the boiling water and stir. Cover and let stand for 10 minutes. Using a fork, separate the grains then add the preserved lemon, parsley, almonds and nigella seeds. Serve on a platter with the kumara chips, if using, on top.

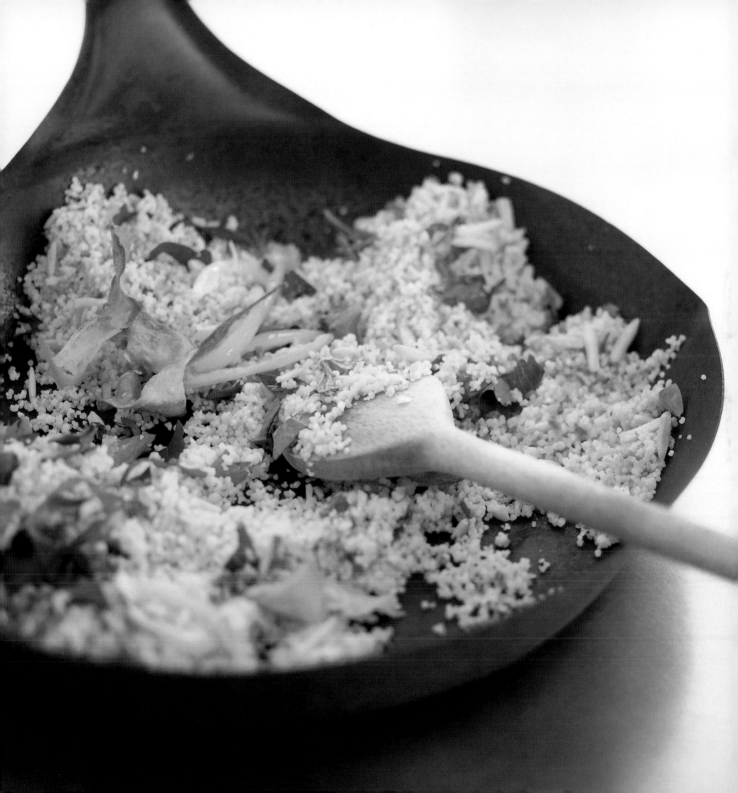

Soups and stews are the 'salads' of winter, the things we crave when it's cold and our bodies are chilled to the bone. What's nicer than coming home at night, our cheeks red from the cold, to tuck into a bowl of hot soup or stew?

During winter it's no surprise that we seem to want to go out less, go to bed earlier and feel nurtured and warm. Respond to your body during the colder months and eat lovely, hot, nurturing and comforting food. Make a big pot of soup, batch it into containers and take it to work for lunch or freeze it to have in the evenings when you've arrived home late and don't feel like cooking. For reluctant or inexperienced cooks, dinner parties can be made simple by preparing a soup or stew in advance and heating it up when the guests are almost ready to sit down.

Experiment with legumes – they offer so much support during winter. Hearty and sustaining, they're also low in fat and terrific for vegetarians who need extra protein in their diet. (Combine them with a grain for a complete protein.)

This section contains some of my favourite recipes – I hope you enjoy them as much as I do.

soups & stews

bean and tomato soup

" This is a variation on the old minestrone, but the pasta has been replaced with a variety of my favourite legumes. This soup is so **thick, satisfying and nourishing**. Put it to the test to see which one keeps you satisfied longer: one day take a bowl of this soup to work for lunch; the next day have a bowl of pumpkin soup. Please don't write to me – I already know the answer! "

2 cups Dina's tomato sauce
   (page 20)

4 cups vegetable stock

1 cup chopped fresh Roma (plum)
   tomatoes

½ red capsicum (bell pepper),
   chopped into small chunks

1 stick celery, roughly chopped

1 small turnip, peeled and roughly
   chopped

3 zucchinis (courgettes), chopped
   into small chunks

about 10 button mushrooms, sliced

1 cup canned or cooked (see page
   177–8) kidney beans

1 cup canned or cooked (see page
   177–8) lima (butter) beans

¼ cup chopped fresh parsley

pitted kalamata olives (optional),
   to taste

serves 6 generously

In a large stockpot heat the tomato sauce and the vegetable stock. Add the chopped vegetables and mushrooms, beans and parsley and bring to the boil. Reduce the heat and simmer for 60 minutes. If using olives, add them in the last 15 minutes of cooking.

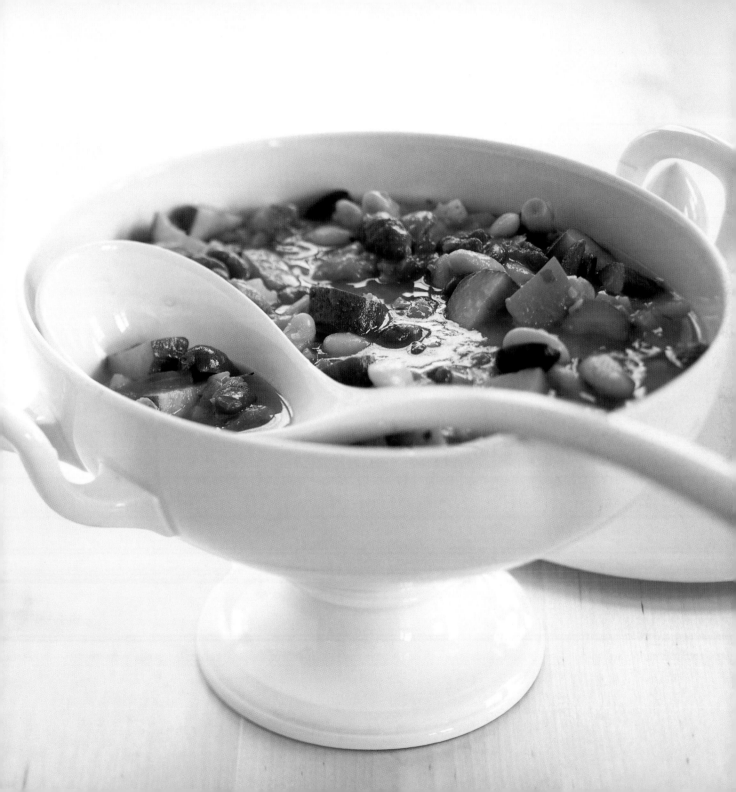

mediterranean fish stew

"With Dina's tomato sauce in the fridge or freezer, you can create a mid-week dinner party in minutes. I tested this recipe on a **friend who is a committed carnivore**; for her, no meal is complete without meat or fish – and she's not very keen on fish because it 'has bones'. This meal worked. Quite unintentionally, my friend was fooled into believing she was eating chicken and, once the true nature of the beast was revealed, she couldn't convince even herself that she didn't like it. "

4 cups Dina's tomato sauce
   (page 20)

juice of 2 oranges

zest of ½ orange

½ cup red wine

2 small bulbs fennel (finocchio), thinly
   sliced

500 g (1 lb) tuna fillets (or any other
   firm, fleshy fish), cut into 2.5 cm
   (1 in) chunks

freshly ground black pepper, to taste

4 servings Italian green salad
   (page 27)

serves 4

Heat the tomato sauce in a large pan with the orange juice, orange zest and red wine. Add the fennel, bring the mixture to the boil, then reduce the heat and simmer for 25 minutes. Drop the fish into the stew, season with pepper and simmer for 2 minutes. Serve immediately with the Italian green salad.

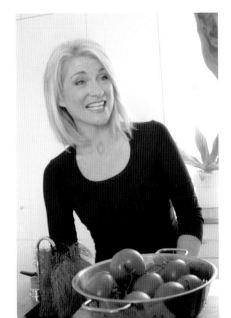

tofu and soba miso soup

" This is a basic recipe for miso soup. Once you have some dashi on hand, all you need is miso and you can play with many variations – with or without noodles, using vegetables of the season – and it will take only minutes. Unlike many other soups, this is much better eaten on the day of making. I give this soup to my clients when they are lacking in energy and feel like they might be fighting an infection. "

1 quantity dashi (page 19)
2 heads bok choy
150 g (5 oz) firm tofu
100 g (3½ oz) buckwheat noodles
   (soba)
2 tablespoons mugi miso
½ sheet nori (dried seaweed), cut into
   2.5 cm (1 in) squares

serves 6

Bring the dashi to the boil. Wash the bok choy, cut into small pieces and add to the dashi with the tofu and noodles. Simmer for 6 minutes or until the noodles are cooked. While the noodles are cooking, add a little of the dashi to the miso in a bowl and mix into a smooth paste. When the noodles are cooked, drop the nori squares into the soup. Stir in the miso paste but *do not* allow the soup to boil. Serve immediately.

leek and carrot soup

"Cock-a-leekie soup is a traditional Scottish dish, which I believe was originally made using a cockerel. Probably because cockerels were not readily available, over the years they came to be replaced by chickens. My mother used to make this soup all the time in winter, as it was an absolute family favourite. This recipe is yet another variation, with both the cockerel and chicken removed. Today I prefer not to eat meat, but this variation seems to provide as much comfort and nourishment as my mother's and helps to remind me of my youth. (If you do want chicken in your soup, add 125 g (4 oz) chopped chicken breast and use 8 cups of chicken stock rather than vegetable stock.) This soup tastes even better the day after making, if you can manage to leave any – it also freezes well."

1 tablespoon olive oil

1 onion, finely chopped

1 small carrot, grated

3 leeks, washed and sliced

50 g (2 oz) long-grain brown rice

8 cups vegetable stock

1 pinch sea salt

freshly ground black pepper, to taste

serves 6

Heat the oil in a large pan and sauté the onion and carrot until the onion is soft. Add the leeks, rice and vegetable stock, and bring to the boil. Once boiled, reduce to a simmer and partially cover the pan. Simmer for 50 minutes then remove from the heat. Season with sea salt and pepper and serve.

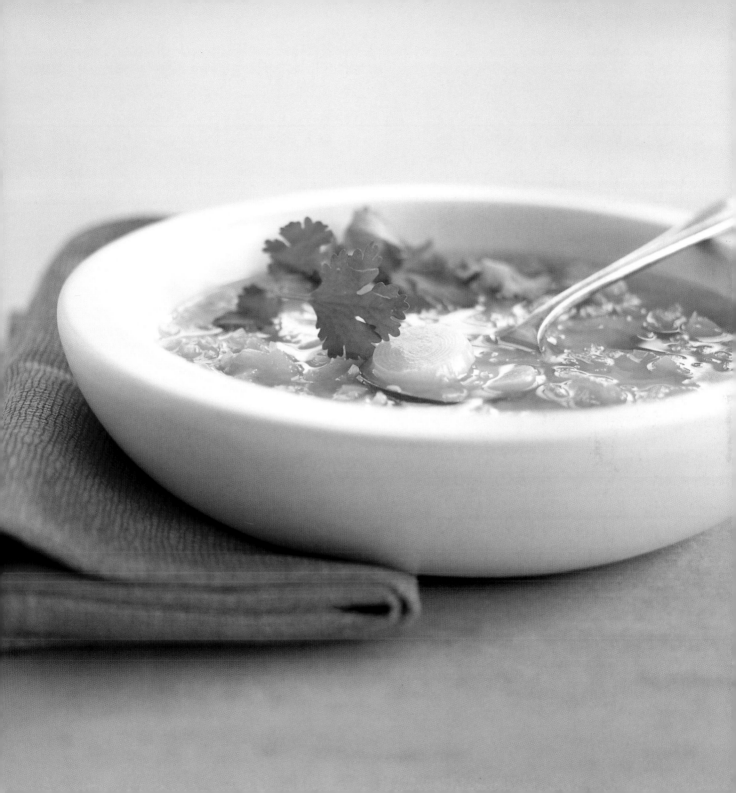

spicy black beans and pancakes with sweetcorn and caper salsa

"The colours, flavours and textures of this meal work beautifully together. This is 'cool', hearty, comforting vegetarian cooking at its best. It's cool because it's so easy – there's no need to get into a flap about the timing of it all. The beans and salsa are even better when made in advance."

fresh coriander (cilantro) sprigs, to serve

natural yoghurt, to serve

6 servings seasoned spinach and
  olive oil (page 27)

beans

1 cup black beans, soaked overnight

6 cups water

1 x 10 cm (4 in) strip kombu

2 teaspoons cumin seeds

1 teaspoon coriander seeds

2 teaspoons mustard seeds

1 tablespoon olive oil

1 onion, finely chopped

3 cloves garlic, crushed

2 red chillies, seeded and finely chopped

2 tablespoons tomato puree

¼ cup water

2 x 400 g (13 oz) cans tomatoes >

To make the spicy black beans, rinse the beans and put in a medium pan with the 6 cups of water and kombu, then bring to the boil. Reduce the heat and simmer for 30 minutes or until the beans are tender. Remove the kombu, drain the beans and set aside.

Dry-roast the cumin, coriander and mustard seeds. Once they start to pop, remove from the heat and grind to a powder with a mortar and pestle or spice grinder. Heat the oil in a large pan and sauté the onion, garlic and chilli until the onion is soft. Add the spices and cook for a further 2 minutes. Add the tomato puree and ¼ cup of water and stir until well combined. Crush the tomatoes, add to the pan with the beans and simmer for 40 minutes until the bean mixture is quite thick and the liquid has been almost completely absorbed. >

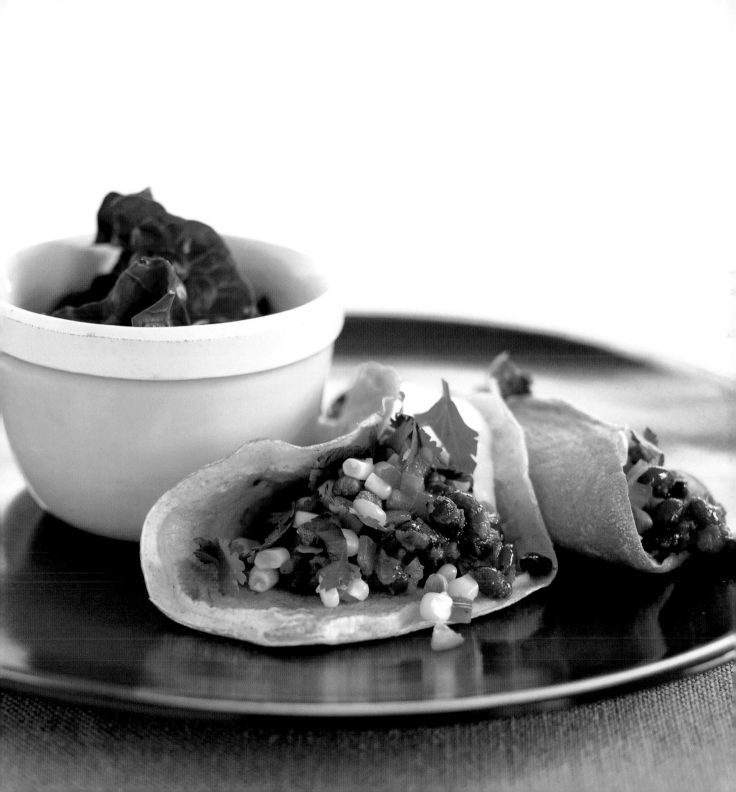

salsa

1 cob (ear) corn

½ red capsicum (bell pepper), finely
   chopped

½ bunch fresh coriander (cilantro),
   finely chopped

2 tablespoons capers (mini capers
   if available), washed and drained

juice of 1 lime

pancakes

⅓ cup chickpea flour

½ cup wholemeal self-raising
   (self-rising) flour

½ teaspoon sea salt

2 small eggs

1¼ cups buttermilk

olive oil, for cooking pancakes

serves 6

While the beans are cooling, prepare the salsa and the pancakes. To make the salsa, steam the corn cob for 3 minutes. Rinse in cold water then cut off the kernels. Mix the capsicum and coriander in a bowl with the corn kernels, capers and lime juice. Refrigerate until ready to serve.

To make the pancakes, sift the flours and salt into a bowl. Make a well in the centre. Beat the eggs and buttermilk together, pour into the well and whisk until bubbles appear on the surface and the batter is free of lumps. Cover the bowl with plastic wrap and set aside for 20 minutes. Pour the batter into a jug. Coat a small non-stick omelette pan with a tiny amount of olive oil and heat. Pour enough batter into the pan to cover the base and wait until bubbles appear on the top of the pancake before flipping to cook the other side. Keep the cooked pancakes warm. Repeat the process until all the batter is used. Spoon the hot beans onto the pancakes, top with salsa and garnish with a spoonful of natural yoghurt and a sprig of coriander. Serve with seasoned spinach and olive oil.

shiitake mushroom soup

"A friend of mine recently received extremely bad news about her health. Coming to terms with the news and a future supported by medication, she lost her appetite and became extremely depressed. The naturally sweet flavour of shiitake mushrooms is very **comforting in such times of stress**. After three days struggling with food, this soup worked a treat for my friend. That evening she regained her appetite and felt calmer than she had in days. But don't think that this soup is only worth eating when you are slightly under the weather – it is delicious, too, and makes a perfect starter for a meal. The soup can be pre-prepared: just heat through and add the cabbage 5 minutes before serving. "

12 dried shiitake mushrooms

8 cups hot water

6 cups cold water

1 x 2.5 cm (1 in) piece ginger, peeled

2 star anise

3 tablespoons mirin

3 tablespoons shoyu (soy sauce)

1 spring onion (scallion), roughly
  chopped

1 carrot, peeled and cut into julienne
  slices

2 cups Chinese cabbage, sliced

½ cup chopped fresh coriander
  (cilantro)

1 spring onion (scallion), extra,
  chopped

serves 4

Soak the shiitake in the hot water for no less than 30 minutes. Rinse the mushrooms, cut off and discard their stalks and slice the caps thinly. Put the cold water in a medium saucepan and add the ginger, star anise, mirin, shoyu and roughly chopped spring onion. Slowly bring to the boil, add the carrot and shiitake and simmer for a further 15 minutes. Add the Chinese cabbage then cook for a further 5 minutes. Remove the ginger and star anise and serve the soup with a garnish of chopped coriander and spring onion.

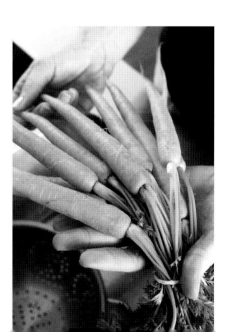

fragrant lentil soup

" Legumes such as lentils are a terrific source of carbohydrate for energy, protein and fibre. They are low in fat and have a low GI. Often neglected as a staple food by our modern, fast-paced society, they are surprisingly easy to prepare. For a variation on this recipe, cook the soup on a very low heat for a further 30–40 minutes until the lentils have virtually disintegrated. Serve over toasted sourdough, avocado and steamed English spinach. "

2 cups red lentils

2 teaspoons olive oil

1 large onion, finely chopped

3 cloves garlic, crushed

1 teaspoon cumin seeds

1 teaspoon coriander seeds

½ teaspoon mustard seeds

½ teaspoon cloves

2 x 400 g (13 oz) cans tomatoes

1 cup kumara (sweet potato), peeled
   and diced

8 cups vegetable stock

sea salt, to taste

1 tablespoon chopped fresh coriander
   (cilantro)

6 tablespoons low-fat natural yoghurt

warmed sourdough or wholegrain
   bread

serves 6

Rinse the lentils in cold water and set aside. Heat the oil in a large non-stick saucepan and sauté the onion and garlic until softened but not brown. Meanwhile, roast the cumin, coriander, mustard seeds and cloves in a dry frying pan until they start to pop. Grind the seeds in a mortar and pestle, add to the onion and garlic and stir for 2 minutes. Add the tomatoes, kumara, vegetable stock and lentils. Bring to the boil then reduce heat and simmer, covered, for 1 hour or until the lentils are tender. Season with salt and serve with chopped coriander, yoghurt and warmed bread.

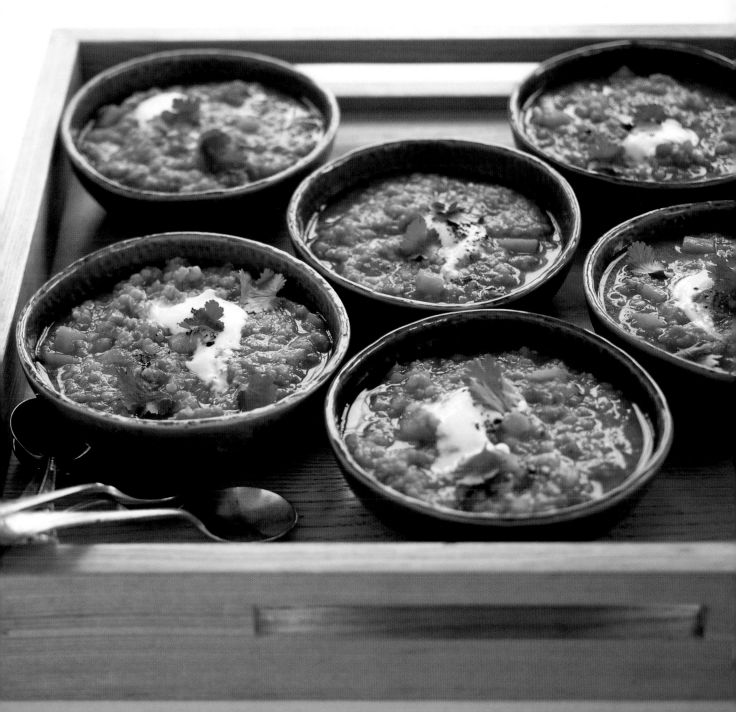

You will notice that I don't insist you go organic with everything. The cost of organic produce is prohibitive for many people, so make it a rule to buy food that's as fresh and as natural as you can. With raw salads, however, buying organic is worth the investment, particularly with tomatoes. Play with dressings, buy seasonal fruit and vegetables and be creative. In summer choose fresh, crisp green leaves and beans, and in winter make a delicious warm salad with roasted root vegetables.

For freshness and nutritional value, I prefer to buy mesclun – a mix of young salad leaves, such as rocket (arugula), endives, baby spinach, watercress, tatsoi and some of the darker greens, which can be quite hot and peppery. Forget cos (romaine) and iceberg lettuce – the leaves may have crunch, but they hold little flavour or nutritional value.

Herbs are an appealing addition to salads. If serving the salad on its own, let the herbs and the strength of the leaves dictate the dressing. If the salad is a side dish, choose a dressing that will work with all the flavours. Experiment with different combinations and have fun!

Here are some good leaf, herb and dressing combinations
- tatsoi and coriander (cilantro) with sesame or Asian dressing
- rocket (arugula), English spinach and basil with a balsamic dressing
- endive with a simple vinaigrette and sea salt or with a miso or flaxseed (linseed) oil dressing

salads

buckwheat noodle, bok choy and pine nut salad

" This salad makes a delicious lunch and can be **made in minutes**. Although best served immediately after cooking, it can also be made in the evening and the leftovers taken to work the next day. It makes a nice change from sandwiches and is a very satisfying high-energy meal that will keep you going for the remainder of the day. " "

2 tablespoons pine nuts

200 g (6½ oz) buckwheat noodles
   (soba)

2 bunches bok choy

4 tablespoons miso dressing
   (page 15)

serves 4

Dry-roast the pine nuts in a small pan until golden and set aside. Bring a large pan of salted water to the boil and add the noodles. Reduce to a simmer and cook for 4 minutes, taking care not to overcook them. Once cooked, rinse them under cold running water to prevent them sticking. Wash the bok choy, trim and roughly chop – don't chop too small or it will overcook. Steam for no more than 2 minutes to ensure that the stalks remain crunchy. Remove from the heat and stir the bok choy through the noodles. Add the dressing and top with the pine nuts.

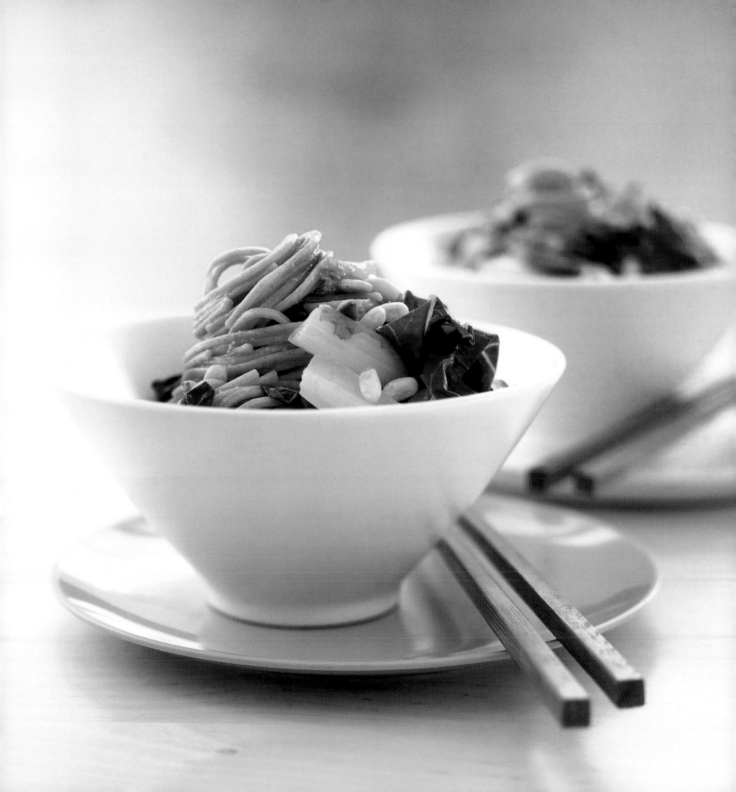

fennel, beetroot leaf and olive salad with brazil nut pesto

"Some authorities say that if a man eats four brazil nuts a day, it helps to **ward off prostate cancer**. I usually find that line helps my male clients to start munching away at these delicious nuts. They can also help ease depression. Don't go overboard with them though, as they are very high in fat. "

1 small bunch endive

1 small bunch beetroot (beet) greens, steamed (page 24)

1 small bulb fennel (finocchio)

20 kalamata olives

4 vine-ripened tomatoes

1 tablespoon balsamic vinegar

pesto

2 cloves garlic

1 cup basil

½ cup olive oil

⅓ cup brazil nuts

2 tablespoons fresh thyme, chopped

juice of 1 lemon

serves 4

To make the pesto, blend all the ingredients in a food processor to form a rough paste.

Wash and dry the endive and mix with the beetroot greens. Trim the fennel and cut into very fine slices. Arrange the mixed leaves and fennel on individual plates and place the olives and tomatoes around. Sprinkle over the balsamic vinegar and top with a spoonful of the pesto.

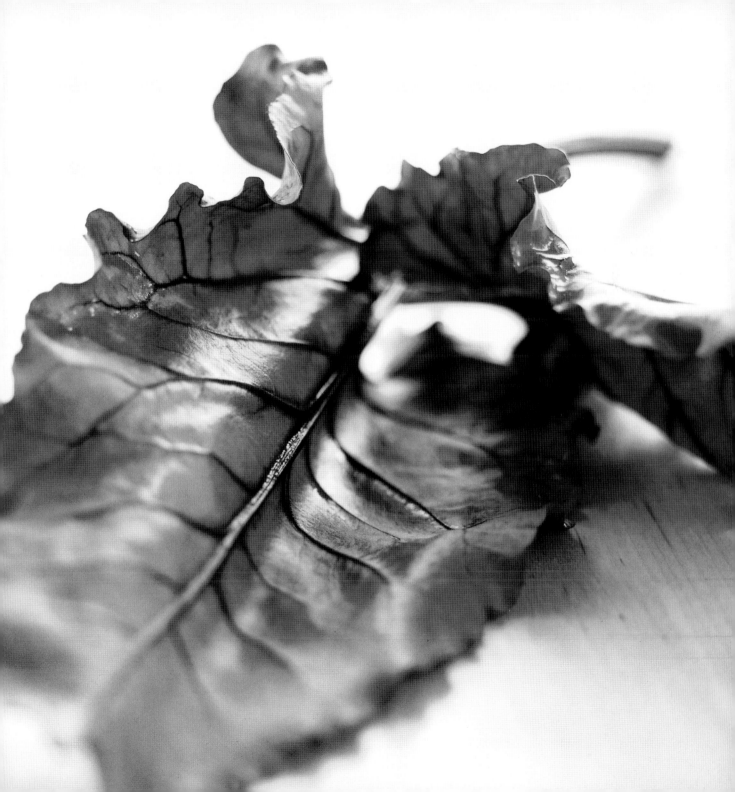

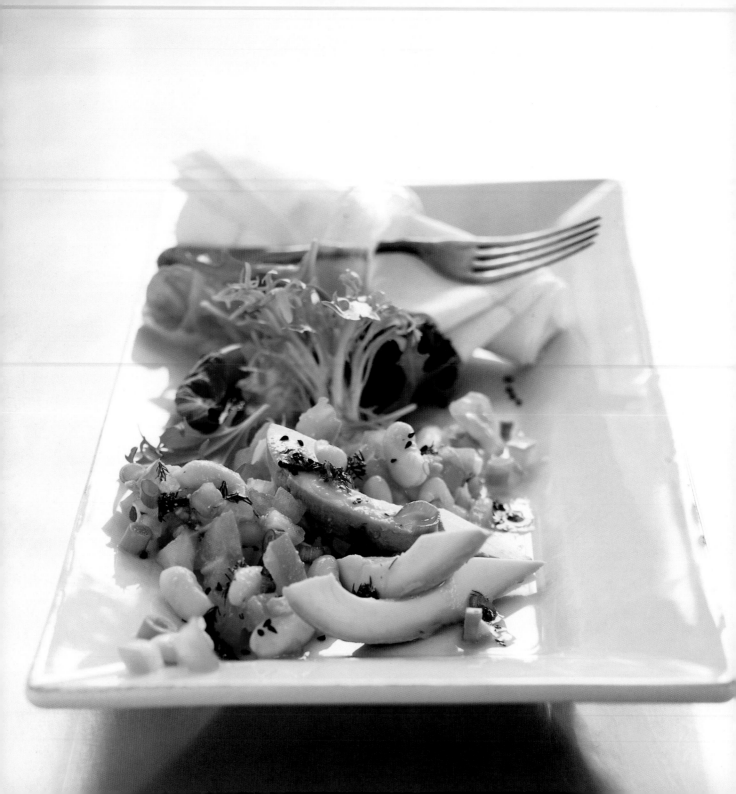

avocado and bean salad

*"*Another 'gate to plate' dish that takes only minutes, particularly when the dressing is already in the fridge and you have a can of haricot (navy) beans. All the same, there is something nice about preparing your own beans, particularly as you can control how much salt goes into them. And thank goodness we've come to recognise the value of certain fats in the diet – how could anyone deny themselves a delicious avocado? This recipe also works well with added salad greens. *"*

1 tablespoon fresh dill, chopped

3 tablespoons miso dressing
(page 15)

2 vine-ripened tomatoes

1 cup canned or cooked (see page 177–8) haricot (navy) beans

3 spring onions (scallions), finely chopped

2 small avocados

2 teaspoons nigella seeds

serves 4

Mix the dill into the miso dressing and refrigerate until you are ready to use. Cut the tomatoes into small cubes, mix with the beans and spring onions and refrigerate for at least 1 hour. Serve the beans on a plate with slices of avocado, a sprinkling of nigella seeds and a drizzle of dressing on top.

beetroot, mango and goat's cheese salad

" I made this salad to take on a picnic with some friends, Des and Jill. Des is definitely a 'don't tell him it's good for him' kind of guy and very set in his ways. If hot food does not arrive at the table piping hot he turns ugly! As I thoroughly enjoy their company, I have managed to overcome the stress of cooking for them by picnicking in the park with cold food and lovely wine. Des described this salad as **'a taste sensation'** and I am still reeling with delight at the compliment. The tartness of the pickles against the sweetness of the mango is really exciting. "

2 tablespoons walnut pieces

12 pieces pickled beetroot (beet)
(page 24)

1 ripe mango, cut into cubes

2 cups beansprouts

⅓ cup goat's cheese (chèvre) or
ricotta cheese

serves 2

Dry-roast the walnut pieces in a frying pan and leave to cool. Mix the beetroot slices and mango cubes together, then arrange on a plate with the beansprouts, goat's cheese or ricotta and the walnuts. Chill before serving. Garnish with some salad greens.

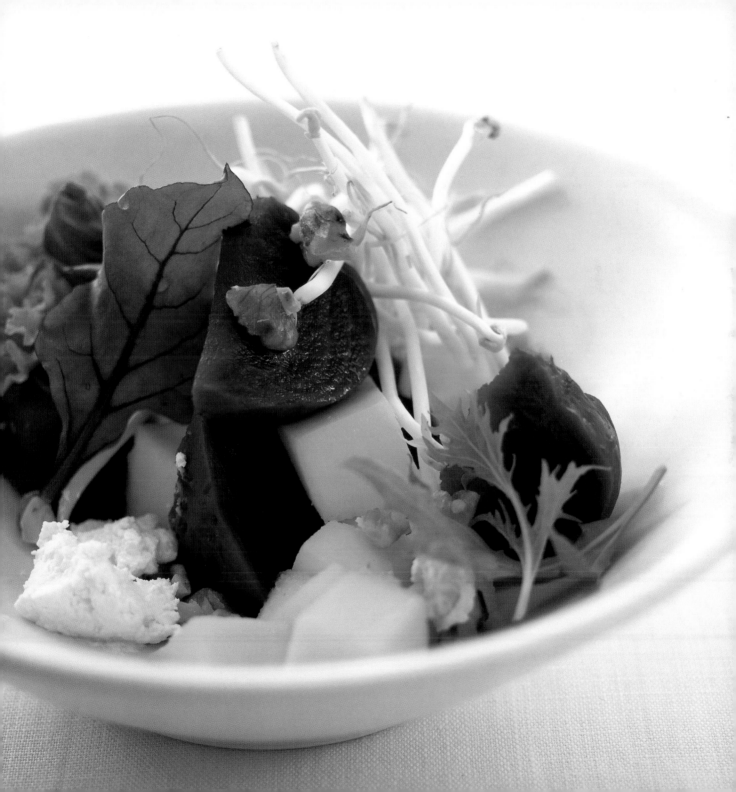

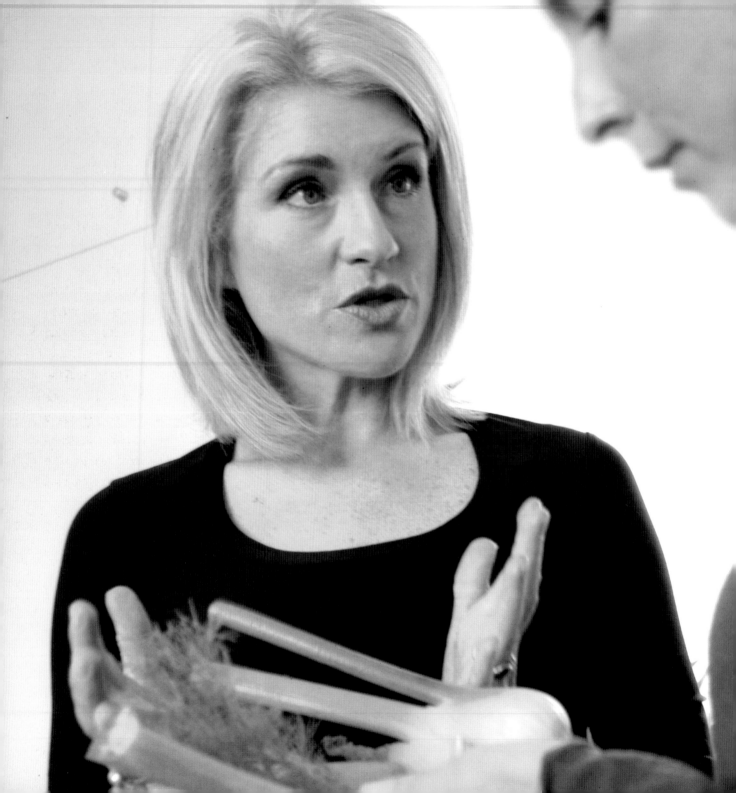

lentil salad

"So many of us suffer from the 4.00 p.m. slump. It's that feeling when you're suddenly so exhausted that you don't think you can go on without coffee and something sweet. The 4.00 p.m. slump is caused by your blood sugar level dropping and your body crying to be picked up. Sweet cakes and biscuits pick you up very quickly, but they drop you down almost as fast. The trick is to eat a lunch that sustains your energy levels into this late afternoon period, so that your body doesn't require more than an apple or a few nuts for an afternoon snack. This lentil salad is a terrific substitute for the lunchtime sandwich. It's packed full of nutrients and just might put an end to the 4.00 p.m. sweet attack. "

½ cup green lentils

2 cups water

1 x 10 cm (4 in) strip kombu

pinch sea salt

2 cloves garlic, shaved into fine slivers

½ red capsicum (bell pepper)

1 vine-ripened tomato

5 mushrooms

½ avocado

4 spring onions (scallions)

2 tablespoons finely chopped rocket
   (arugula)

½ tablespoon balsamic vinegar

½ tablespoon olive oil

1 tablespoon finely chopped fresh mint

cracked black pepper, to taste

serves 2

Soak the lentils overnight, then drain and put in a pot with the water and the kombu strip and bring to the boil. Once boiling, remove the kombu and reduce the heat to a simmer. (If you don't remove the kombu before you serve this salad, it will be inedible, as my sister discovered when she tested this recipe!) Simmer for 20 minutes then add the sea salt. Simmer for a further 5 minutes or until the lentils are tender. Drain and rinse the lentils in cold water and set aside to cool. In a dry frying pan, roast the garlic shavings until they are brown and deliciously fragrant. Finely chop the capsicum, tomato, mushrooms, avocado and spring onions, then mix with the lentils and rocket. Combine the balsamic vinegar, olive oil and mint and pour over the salad. Serve with the shaved garlic and cracked black pepper on top.

root vegetable salad

" I like this salad served with a strongly flavoured soft goat's cheese, but it works just as well with fish or lamb. It's a **perfect winter lunch** when you have guests coming over and don't want to be a slave in the kitchen. The dressing can be prepared in advance and the rest is simple. "

3 medium-sized carrots, peeled

½ medium-sized kumara (sweet potato), peeled

6 new potatoes

10 shallots

4 zucchinis (courgettes)

2 cloves garlic

2 tablespoons olive oil

sea salt, to taste

½ bunch rocket (arugula)

dressing

2 teaspoons cumin seeds

1 x 2.5 cm (1 in) piece preserved lemon (page 16)

5 tablespoons fresh mint, finely chopped

3 tablespoons white wine vinegar

3 tablespoons olive oil

½ teaspoon honey

serves 4

Preheat the oven to 190°C (375 °F, Gas Mark 4). Cut the carrots into large, long chunks. The kumara and new potatoes should be cut into pieces of roughly the same size (about 2.5 cm (1 in) cubes). Peel the shallots but leave them whole. Trim the ends of the zucchinis and cut into quarters. Peel the garlic and slice very finely. Put the olive oil in a roasting tin and heat in the oven for about 3 minutes. Remove the tin from the oven and add all the vegetables in one layer, tossing them in the hot oil to coat. Season with sea salt, return the pan to the oven and roast for 40 minutes, turning the vegetables occasionally.

To make the dressing, dry-roast the cumin seeds in a pan then grind to a fine powder with a mortar and pestle. Using a fork, mash the preserved lemon and mix it in a bowl with all the other dressing ingredients. The dressing is not meant to be runny, so don't panic – you haven't done anything wrong!

Once the vegetables are cooked, immediately toss through the rocket leaves so they wilt, then add the dressing.

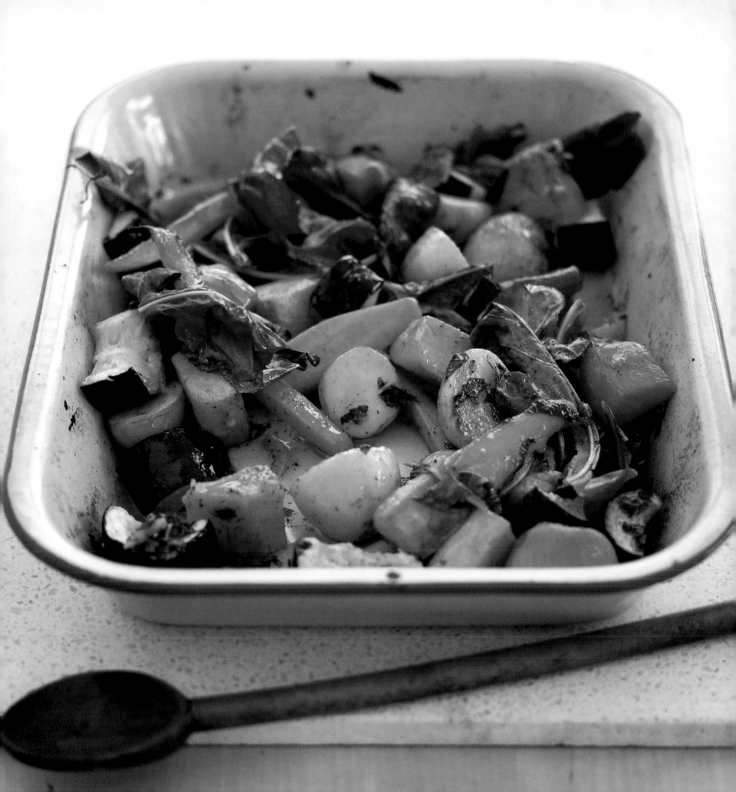

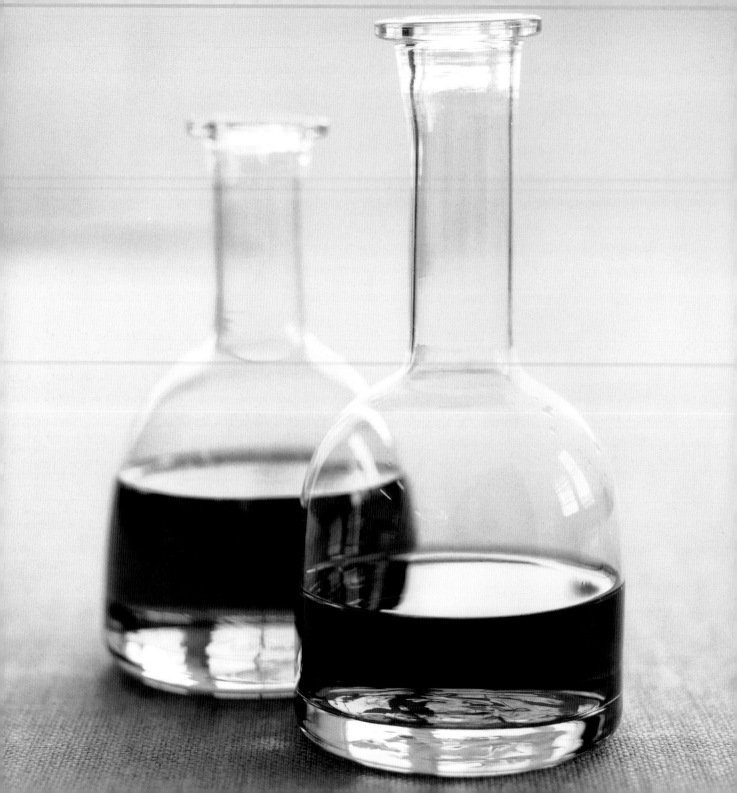

rocket, basil and avocado salad with nigella seeds

❝ When I first picked up a jar of nigella seeds (often incorrectly called black cumin seeds), accompanying them was a leaflet that listed the many healing properties of these miraculous little gems. According to the leaflet, and a little further research on my part, they help hay fever, headaches, hair loss, asthma, a feeling of being rundown, even laziness. Some would say there's nothing they can't cure. Even if it's only half true, I say they taste great, they're good for you, so go for it. You'll often see them baked on top of Turkish bread – they have a lovely, unusual flavour that I'm completely incapable of describing. ❞

1 tablespoon nigella seeds

1 large bunch baby rocket (arugula)

½ cup fresh basil leaves, loosely
   packed

4 tablespoons olive oil

1 tablespoon white wine vinegar

juice of ½ lime

pinch sea salt

1 avocado, sliced

lemon slices, to serve

za'tar (page 15), to serve

olive oil, to serve

serves 4

Dry-roast the nigella seeds in a pan until fragrant. Set aside to cool. Wash and dry the rocket and basil leaves. Mix the oil, vinegar and lime juice together with the sea salt. Arrange the salad leaves on a flat platter with the slices of avocado on top. Sprinkle the dressing over the salad and top with the nigella seeds. Serve with slices of lemon, a liberal sprinkling of za'tar and olive oil.

spicy red cabbage with apples

" You might be surprised to hear that I am **a bit of a traditionalist** when it comes to food on certain occasions. I don't usually eat meat, but on Christmas Day, if I'm in Scotland with the family, there can be nothing other than turkey, oatmeal stuffing, roast potatoes, carrots, Brussels sprouts, cranberry sauce and gravy. Unless this exact combination is served, for me the meal is as good as ruined. Imagine my horror when my sister, Jennifer, introduced Delia Smith's spiced sautéed red cabbage with cranberries to the Christmas repertoire. While it was 100 per cent banned from ever again making an appearance on 25 December, the dish had distinct possibilities, so I have created this version, which is quite delicious. "

1 tablespoon corn oil

1 large clove garlic, finely chopped

1 Spanish (red) onion, finely chopped

½ teaspoon ground cinnamon

½ teaspoon ground nutmeg

2.5 cm (1 in) piece ginger, grated

¼ red cabbage, cored and finely shredded

1½ tablespoons organic apple cider vinegar

1 tablespoon apple concentrate

pinch sea salt

freshly ground black pepper, to taste

1 green apple, grated with skin on

¼ cup walnuts, chopped

serves 6 as a side salad

In a very large heavy-based pan or wok, heat the oil and sauté the garlic, onion, spices and ginger for 3 minutes. Once the onion is cooked, increase the heat, add the cabbage and toss continually to coat in the oil and spices. Reduce the heat to low and add the apple cider vinegar and apple concentrate. Cook for another 6 minutes, season, then remove from the heat – the cabbage should still be crunchy. Stir through the grated apple and walnuts and serve immediately.

Serve spicy red cabbage with apples with

- cold turkey breast
- grilled chicken
- pork fillets

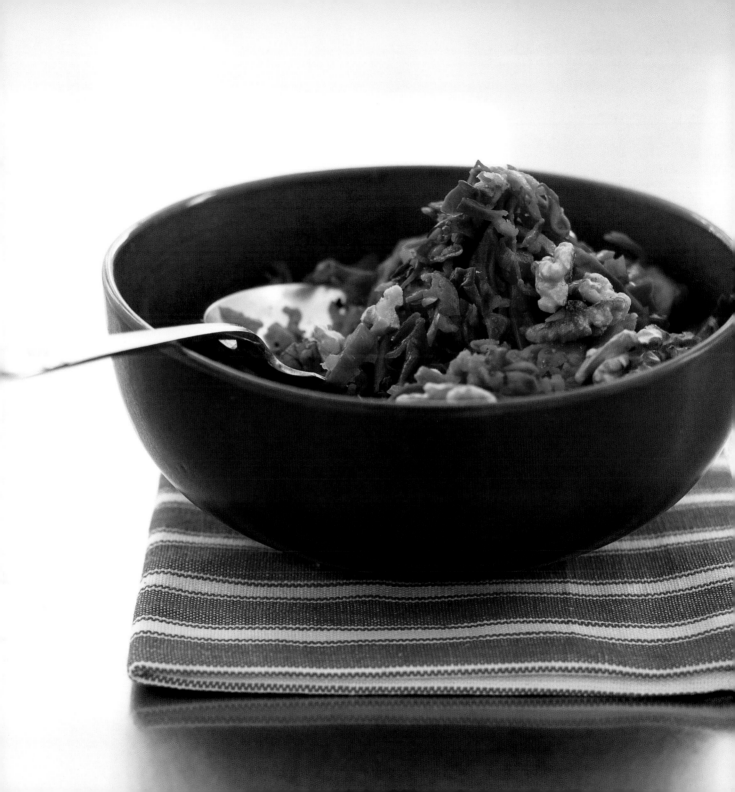

sesame, noodle and sprout salad

> " This is a lovely salad to **serve with a barbecue of fish or chicken**, or on its own for lunch. I have also packed it into small noodle boxes and served them as party food. " "

½ red capsicum (bell pepper), cut into
   strips
½ large carrot, cut into strips
2 heads bok choy, washed, trimmed
   and chopped
100 g (3 oz) buckwheat noodles
1 tablespoon chopped fresh mint
2 tablespoons chopped fresh
   coriander (cilantro)
2 teaspoons finely chopped lemongrass
2 cups beansprouts

dressing
2 tablespoons tahini
3 tablespoons sesame oil
3 tablespoons rice vinegar
2 tablespoons water
1 tablespoon fish sauce
1 teaspoon seeded and finely
   chopped fresh red chilli

serves 6

In a bamboo steamer, steam the capsicum and carrot for about 3 minutes each and the bok choy for about 2 minutes – take care not to overcook them. When steamed, rinse the vegetables in cold water and drain thoroughly. Boil the noodles until soft and tender (about 4 minutes) then drain and rinse in cold water. Mix the steamed vegetables with the noodles, herbs and beansprouts.

To make the dressing, shake the tahini and sesame oil in a jar until thoroughly combined. Add the remaining ingredients and shake vigorously until well combined. The dressing can be refrigerated until ready to use. Pour the dressing over the salad and serve.

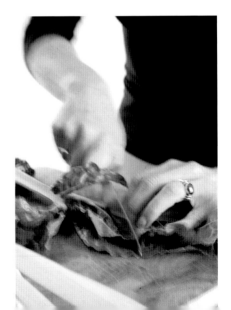

beetroot, orange and walnut salad

"I made this salad for a girls' lunch in honour of our friend Philippa, who was getting married the next day. While we were thrilled that she was getting married, after the wedding she was leaving the country, which was sad for all of us. Phil was emotional, as brides usually are, and so were we, as girlfriends usually are. Lunch therefore had to be easily digested, light, and soothing for our delicate states. Soft, sweet foods, fresh vegetables and oats are **wonderful foods for anxiety**. I'm not very good at measuring quantities of greens – I always get excited and buy too much. When I am preparing a salad for four, I buy about four small handfuls from the mixed salad section, such as endive, rocket (arugula) and watercress."

¼ cup walnuts

4 handfuls mixed greens

3 medium-sized roast beetroot (beet)
   (page 23), cut into 2.5 cm (1 in)
   pieces

1 orange, peeled

⅓ cup soft goat's cheese (chèvre)

1 tablespoon olive oil

dressing

2 tablespoons olive oil

2 tablespoons walnut oil

2 tablespoons apple cider vinegar

1 teaspoon honey

1 teaspoon grated orange zest

serves 4

Mix the dressing ingredients together in a jar. Break the walnuts into small pieces and dry-roast over a medium heat, taking care not to burn them. Set aside. Wash the salad greens, arrange on four plates and place the beetroot on top. Cut the orange into small segments and place in the centre of the plate with the walnuts on top. Place small pieces of goat's cheese between the beetroot pieces, divide the dressing among the plates and drizzle with olive oil.

king prawn and mango salsa salad

❝ I feel a bit of a fraud writing up this recipe; it is so old and tried and tested, with hundreds of variations in virtually every cookbook you open. It's just that every time I give the recipe to a client they love it and they **cook it up constantly**. On the 'yum-o-meter' it rates very highly, but what's even better is that it is truly the quickest, easiest and most elegant dish to put together. If the budget is a bit tight, chargrill a piece of chicken breast in place of the prawns (shrimp) – it works just as well. This meal is definitely a treat and should not be made too often. Prawns are a good source of protein, but have quite high cholesterol levels; therefore, eat them in moderation please! **❞**

16 fresh cooked king prawns (jumbo
   shrimp)
juice of 2 limes
4 small handfuls mixed rocket
   (arugula) and English spinach leaves
1 large mango, cut into small cubes
½ Spanish (red) onion, finely chopped
1 small red chilli, seeded and finely
   chopped
1 cup chopped fresh coriander
   (cilantro)
2 small avocados, sliced
cracked black pepper, to taste
fresh coriander (cilantro) sprigs,
   to serve

serves 4

Shell and devein the prawns and sprinkle with half the lime juice. Wash and dry the salad leaves. To make the mango salsa, mix the mango, Spanish onion, chilli, coriander and remaining lime juice in a bowl. Arrange the salad greens on a plate, spoon over the mango salsa and top with slices of avocado and the king prawns. Top with the pepper and garnish each serving with a sprig of coriander.

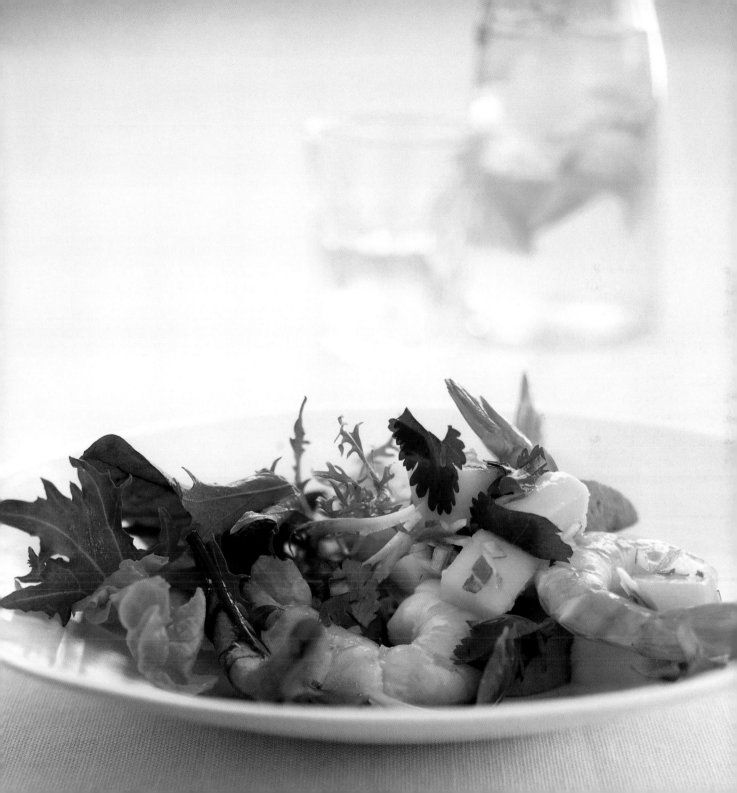

Did you have a teacher at school who was so inspiring that the subject he or she taught became your favourite – a subject most children typically loathed, like maths or physics? I would love to inspire people to love tofu and vegetables. Tofu is handy if you're busy. Keep a block in the fridge at all times – it's a great fallback when the cupboards and fridge are all but bare . . . bare of everything except some vibrant vegetables.

No main meal should be brought to the table without vegetables. Focus mainly on the greens, then those with the lovely bright colours and pay less attention to the plain, bland, white vegetables like potatoes or parsnip. Vegetables should never be an afterthought. I'm always amazed when my clients go for a week without a single vegetable passing their lips. And yet vegetables can take minutes to prepare, and 'maketh the meal'.

vegetables & tofu

spinach and mushroom roll

" It's very exciting making this roll for the first time. You'll **feel like a master chef** pulling this impressive creation from the oven. The contrasting flavours of tomato and goat's cheese work so well together and complement the earthier flavours of silver beet and mushroom. **""**

1 bunch silver beet (Swiss chard),
   washed and stalks removed

½ teaspoon ground nutmeg

¼ cup soft goat's cheese (chèvre)

cracked black pepper, to taste

6 egg whites

1 tablespoon corn oil

2 cups button mushrooms, sliced

1 cup Dina's tomato sauce (page 20)

2–4 servings Italian green salad
   (page 27)

serves 4 as a starter or 2 as a main

Preheat the oven to 180°C (350°F, Gas Mark 4). Cook the silver beet in boiling salted water for 2 minutes. Plunge into cold water, squeeze dry, then blend in a food processor. Stir through the nutmeg, fold in the goat's cheese, then season with pepper and set aside. In a glass or stainless steel bowl, beat the egg whites until they are stiff and form peaks. Fold into the silver beet mixture, being careful not to over-mix, then spread evenly across a baking sheet lined with baking paper. Bake for 20–30 minutes, until cooked through but still soft and springy to the touch.

While the spinach roll is still cooking, heat the corn oil in a small pan and sauté the mushrooms until they are soft. Add the tomato sauce and heat through. Ease the roll from the baking paper using a flat knife and spatula. Put it on a clean tea towel and lay the mushrooms and sauce over the top, leaving the edges clear. Carefully roll it up and serve warm with Italian green salad.

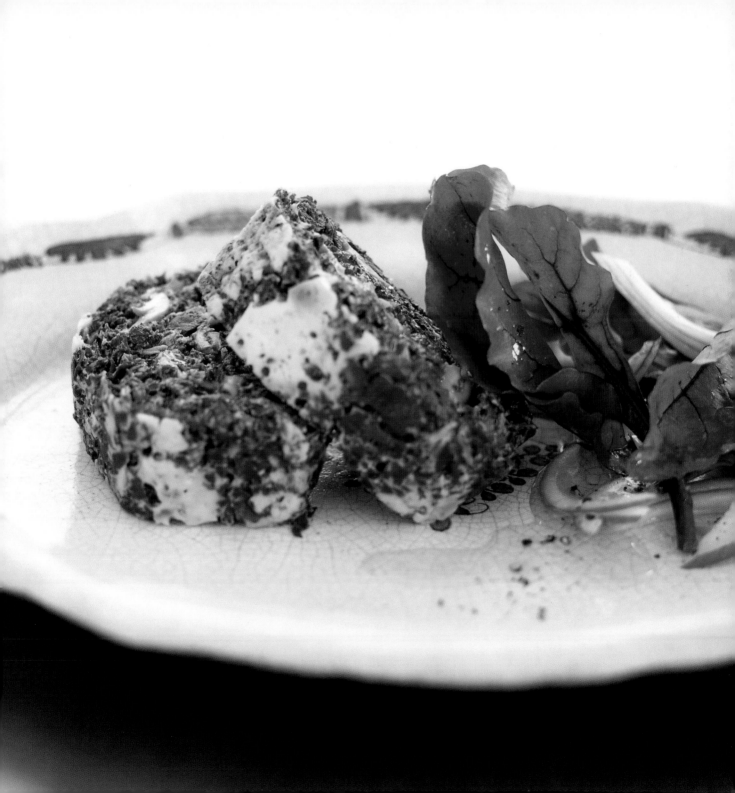

savoury tofu

"This could be described as the **vegetarian equivalent of a meat loaf**. It's warm, comforting and extremely flavoursome. Savoury tofu can also be served cold with salad the next day. 99

500 g (1 lb) firm tofu

2 tablespoons olive oil

3 cloves garlic

1 x 5 cm (2 in) piece ginger,
   peeled and sliced

½ cup water

¼ cup tamari

¼ cup fresh basil

4 servings stir-fried Asian greens
   (page 28)

serves 4

Preheat the oven to 180°C (350°F, Gas Mark 4). Cut the tofu into 1 cm (½ in) slices and brush with the olive oil. Bake on an oven tray for 20–30 minutes until golden brown. Puree the garlic, ginger, water, tamari and basil in a blender or food processor. Marinate the baked tofu in the mixture for up to 1 hour. Drain and return to the oven for 10 minutes then turn the slices and bake for a further 10 minutes. Serve with the stir-fried Asian greens.

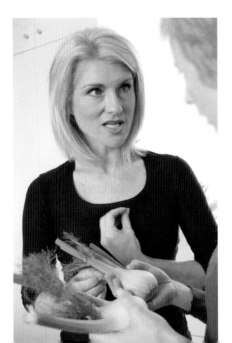

lemon soy cutlets

"I've mentioned Des already – you may remember him: he's the one who won't touch a legume and must have his food served piping hot. His partner, Jill, is a good friend of mine and her attention to detail made her a perfect recipe tester for this book. As a consequence, Des was part of the deal and, despite my initial misgivings, he turned out to be one of the best contributors to this book. I'm sure there was many a night when Jill had to drag him to the table for dinner, but for the most part he was prepared to give the recipes a go. The final recipe on their testing schedule was for these lemon soy cutlets. Jill asked me over that night, I suspect because she had decided that serving Des tofu cutlets would be a battle hard to win on her own. It was music to my ears when Jill asked him if he would eat them again and he responded (in a surprised voice), 'Definitely. Yes.' This meal is very simple but really tasty (just ask Des!). It's a perfect mid-week dinner when you arrive home to a fridge that is bare save for a block of tofu and some salad greens."

250 g (8 oz) firm tofu, drained and cut
   into 1 cm (½ in) slices

2 cloves garlic, crushed

juice of 1 lemon

2 tablespoons shoyu (soy sauce) –
   or tamari, if preferred

1 teaspoon rice syrup – or honey,
   if preferred

¼ cup polenta (cornmeal)

2 teaspoons olive oil

2 servings Asian salad (page 26)

serves 2

Boil the tofu slices in a pan of water until they float to the surface (about 3 minutes). While the tofu is boiling, mix together the garlic, lemon juice, shoyu and rice syrup. Drain the tofu and pat the slices dry with a dry, clean cloth. Pour the garlic mixture over the tofu, turning the slices over so they absorb the flavours of the marinade. Leave the tofu in the marinade for up to 4 hours (but 20 minutes is fine if you're short of time). Dip the tofu into the polenta and coat each side evenly. Heat the oil in a shallow frying pan. Working in batches, drop the cutlets into the pan and fry for 4 minutes on each side or until golden. Repeat until all the cutlets are cooked. Serve with the Asian salad.

balsamic onion, olive and tomato tart

" Serve this delicious tart with lashings of green salad – it **looks and tastes stunning** with the contrasting colours and flavours. The tart filling works particularly well with the coarse-textured oat pastry. "

4 vine-ripened Roma (plum) tomatoes,
 quartered lengthways

1 tablespoon olive oil

2 medium-sized Spanish (red) onions,
 thinly sliced

2 tablespoons balsamic vinegar

1 tablespoon water

1 teaspoon rice syrup

1 wholemeal and oat pastry shell
 (page 22)

⅓ cup pitted olives, halved

⅓ cup fresh basil leaves, torn into
 strips

½ cup soft goat's cheese (chèvre)

6 servings Italian green salad
 (page 27)

serves 6

Preheat the oven to 180°C (350°F, Gas Mark 4). Place the tomatoes on a baking tray lined with baking paper. Brush lightly with the olive oil and bake for 40–50 minutes. While the tomatoes are roasting, put the onions in a pan with the balsamic vinegar, water and rice syrup. Bring to a boil over a medium heat before reducing the heat and simmering until the onions are very soft, tender and sweet. When the tomatoes are cooked, reduce the oven to 150°C (300°F, Gas Mark 2). Line the bottom of the pastry shell with the onions. Arrange the olives on top, then cover with the roasted tomatoes, basil and goat's cheese. Warm in the oven for 10 minutes and serve with the Italian green salad.

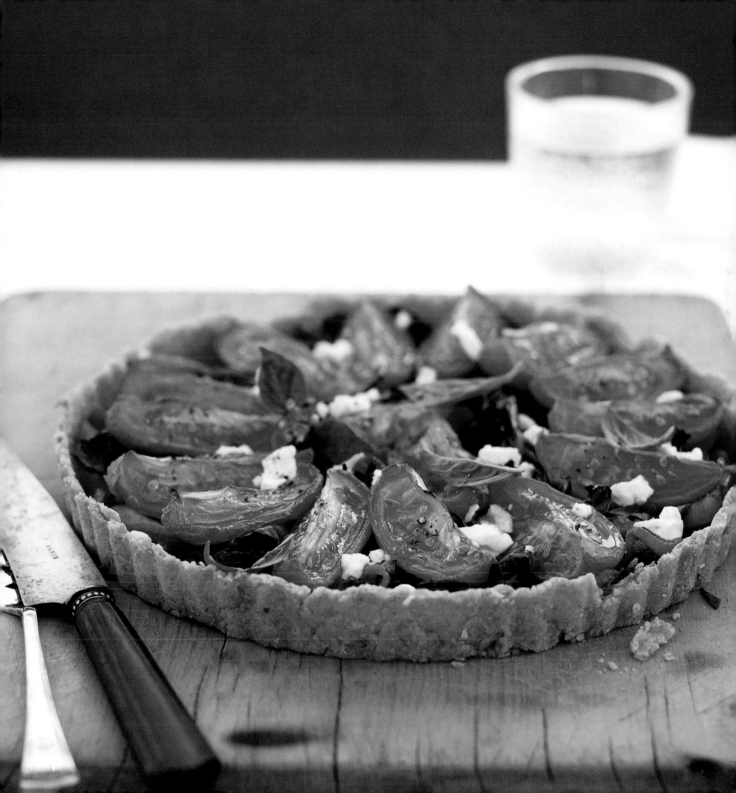

east meets west

"I can't for the life of me think of a name for this dish that will inspire anyone to make it. Certainly, the words 'Brussels sprouts' would send most running for cover, but you have to believe me when I tell you that this dish tastes good. It's also very easy. The truth is that it was created one night when the **cupboards were almost bare** and an unexpected visitor popped in. I liked it, he said he liked it and, when his plate was empty, he asked me what it was called. 'I've no idea,' I replied. 'I'll give it a name when it goes in my book.'"

¼ cup mirin

¼ cup shoyu (soy sauce)

1 medium-sized kumara (sweet potato), peeled and cut into 2.5 cm (1 in) cubes

1 cup tofu, cubed

¼ cup raw cashews

1 cup halved Brussels sprouts

120 g (4 oz) buckwheat noodles

1 tablespoon corn oil

½ tablespoon olive oil

cracked black pepper, to taste

serves 2

Mix the mirin and shoyu together in a bowl. Boil the kumara and tofu in water until the tofu rises to the top and the kumara is just tender. Drain, blot dry and coat in the mirin and shoyu mixture. Dry-roast the cashews in a large frying pan and set aside. Steam the Brussels sprouts for 3 minutes or until they are *just* tender. Boil the noodles for 3–4 minutes or until tender. Heat the corn oil in same pan you used to roast the cashews. Cut the sprouts in half and fry them, cut-side down, until they turn golden. Heat the olive oil in a wok and stir-fry the tofu and kumara until golden. Drain the noodles and stir through the tofu and kumara. Serve in bowls with the Brussels sprouts and roast cashews on top. Season with black pepper.

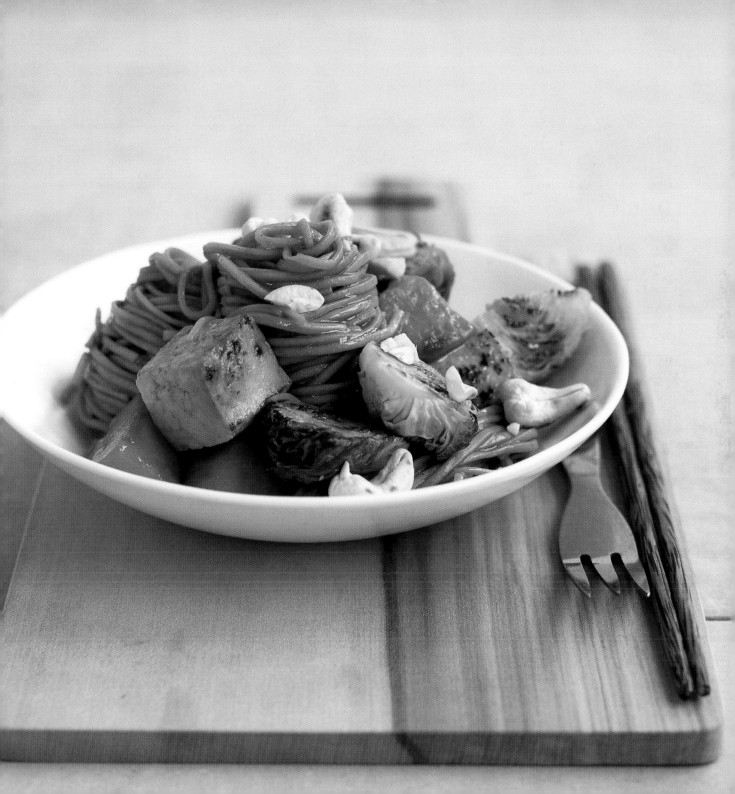

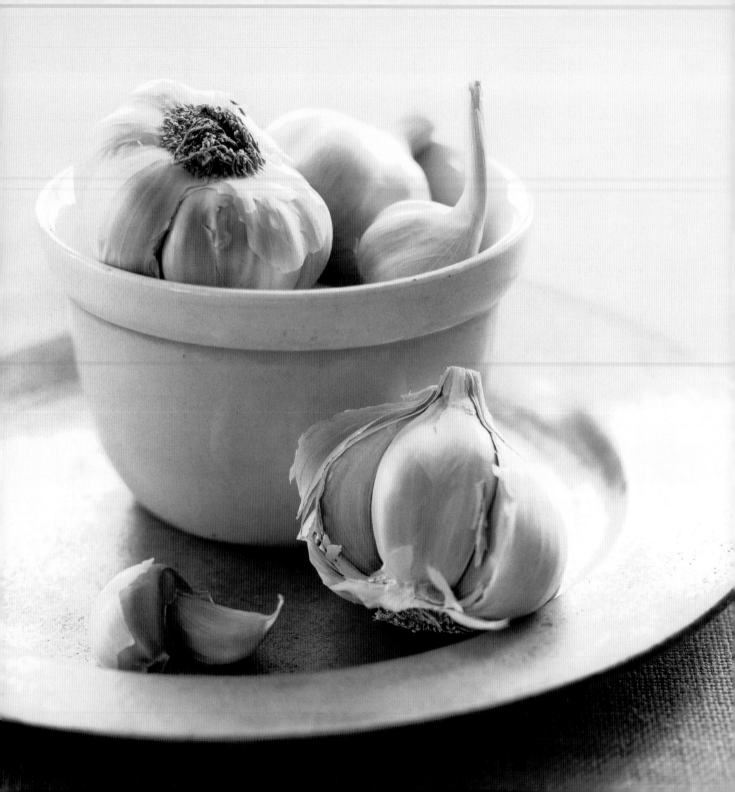

vegetable and pesto tart

" Making this tart is as **simple as making a sandwich**. Make a basic oat pastry shell, fill it with chargrilled vegetables and top with pesto sauce. It couldn't be simpler. Once the pesto is made you can use it with many other things. Just store it in a jar in the fridge with some lemon and olive oil squeezed over the top. It will keep for 3–4 days. **""**

2 zucchinis (courgettes), cut into
    small chunks

2 cups halved button mushrooms

6 Roma (plum) tomatoes, halved

1 tablespoon olive oil

1 wholemeal and oat pastry shell
    (page 22)

pesto

2 cloves garlic, crushed

1 cup (tightly packed) fresh basil leaves

½ cup fresh green peas (I sometimes
    cheat and use frozen)

¼ cup olive oil

1½ tablespoons silken tofu

1½ tablespoons pine nuts,
    dry-roasted

1½ tablespoons walnuts

1 level tablespoon mugi miso

1 tablespoon lemon juice (to stop
    discoloration)

serves 6

To make the pesto, combine all the ingredients in a blender and blend until almost smooth, leaving enough texture in the sauce to make it interesting.

Preheat the oven to 160°C (325°F, Gas Mark 3). Brush the zucchinis, mushrooms and tomatoes lightly with the olive oil then roast for 20 minutes. Turn the oven down to 150°C (300°F, Gas Mark 2). Spread the pesto over the base of the pastry shell, layer the vegetables on top, cover with foil and heat through in the oven for 20 minutes.

baked mushrooms and spinach with sesame sauce

"Take two large, flat field mushrooms, brush off any earth or peel off the skin and treat them as you might a piece of meat or fish. They make the perfect base for a meal. Brush them with olive oil and bake or grill them. Stuff them with yummy fillings or serve them on their own. Make them the focus of the plate and experiment around them. This recipe is an all-time favourite of mine (and of most of my clients). Add sesame sauce and spinach to the dish and the **plate erupts with nutritional goodness.**"

4 large field mushrooms

1 tablespoon olive oil

½ tablespoon sesame seeds

1 bunch English spinach

sauce

½ cup dashi (page 19)

½ cup tahini

2 tablespoons tamari

2 teaspoons maple syrup

1 teaspoon sesame oil

serves 4 as a starter or 2 as a main

Preheat the oven to 180°C (350°F, Gas Mark 4). Break off the mushroom stalks then brush the caps lightly with the olive oil. Place on a baking tray and bake for 20 minutes.

While the mushrooms are baking, prepare the spinach and the sesame sauce. Wash the spinach and remove the lower ends of the stalks. Steam for 3 minutes or until wilted. Once the spinach is cool enough to handle (but not cold), squeeze out all the excess moisture by rolling in a bamboo mat, or pressing in a sieve. To make the sauce, combine all the ingredients in a small saucepan over a low heat until they are warm and thoroughly mixed. Dry-roast the sesame seeds over a low heat and set aside.

Put a piece of rolled-up spinach on each mushroom, pour a tablespoon of the sesame sauce over the top and sprinkle with the sesame seeds.

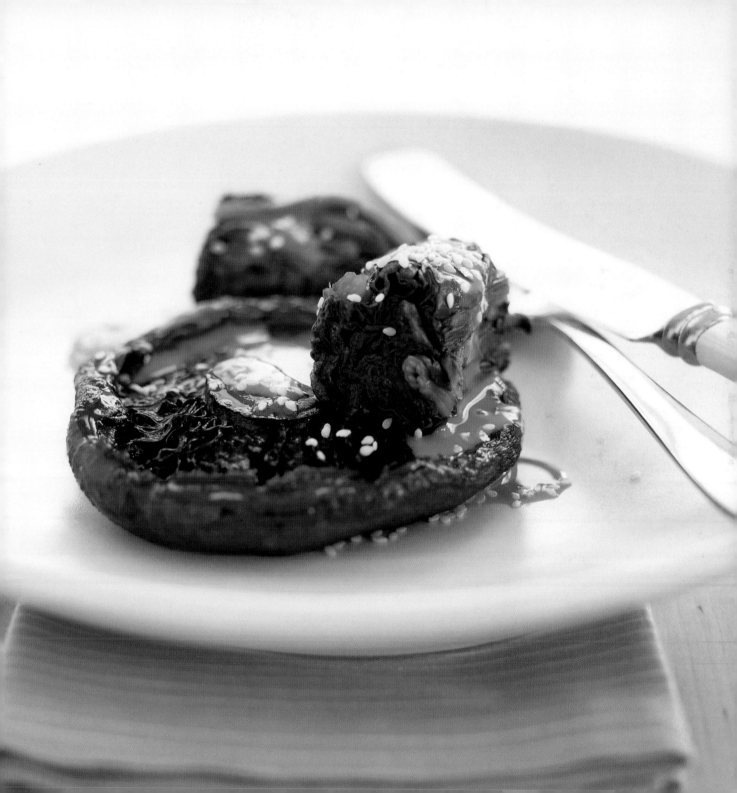

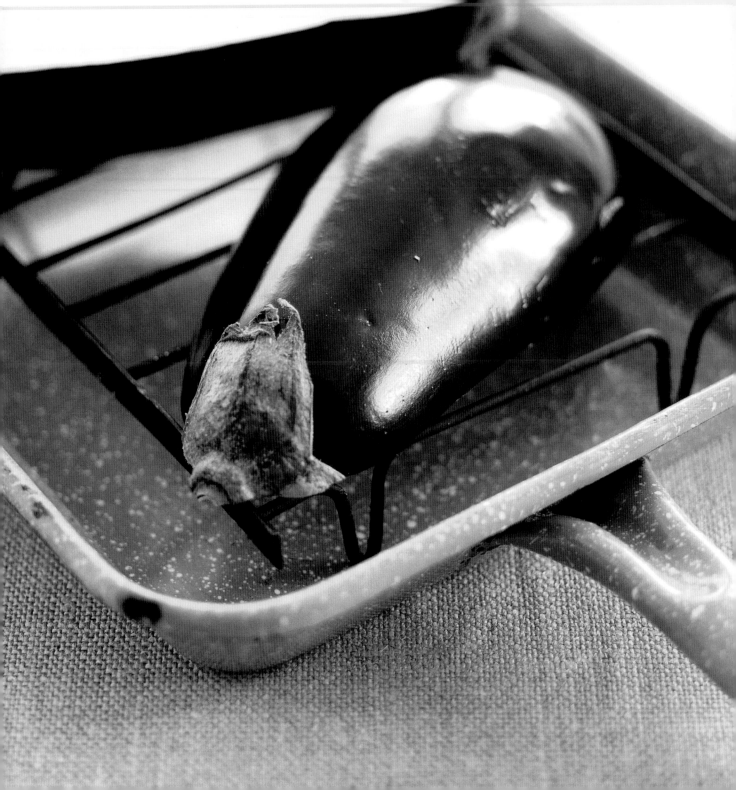

japanese eggplant

66 Often, less is more, which is certainly the case with this **delicious and very simple** eggplant dish. It's so easy to make, but when combined with the sauce no-one would guess that the hardest part was creating sufficient space between the grill-pan and the heat to fit the fruit (yes, it's a fruit, not a vegetable). Serve it with grilled bonito if you want to feel particularly 'Japanesey', or as an accompaniment to lamb or lemon soy cutlets (page 109). If you do serve this dish with white fish or tofu, add another colour to the plate with some greens, to make it more visually appealing. The marinated watercress (page 30) would work splendidly, as would bundles of steamed English spinach. 99

1 eggplant (aubergine)

2 tablespoons shoyu (soy sauce)

1 tablespoon dashi (page 19)

1 x 2.5 cm (1 in) piece ginger, grated

serves 4

Grill (broil) the eggplant whole under a hot grill (broiler) until it feels soft under the skin. Remove and plunge into cold water. Once cool to the touch, quickly peel off the skin and tear the flesh into strips with your hands. Combine the shoyu and dashi, stir in the ginger and pour over the eggplant.

kumara, apple and onion tart

"This tart is a variation on a very unhealthy recipe I once found in a cookbook. The combination of flavours was very interesting so here is a healthier version. Served with Asian salad it's really delicious. It's not a 'gate to plate' recipe but, it's **fun to make**, so I've included it in the book and suggest you make it on a rainy weekend when you feel like being creative and spending time in the kitchen. **"**

1 tablespoon olive oil

2 onions, finely sliced

3 cloves garlic, crushed

1 tablespoon chopped fresh rosemary

1 tablespoon chopped fresh thyme

500 g (1 lb) kumara (sweet potato)

½ tablespoon apple concentrate

½ tablespoon corn oil

½ cup silken tofu

sea salt, to taste

cracked black pepper, to taste

1 sour green apple

1 basic pastry shell (page 22), made
with 1 cup wholemeal flour and
¾ cup chickpea flour

1 teaspoon nigella seeds

6 servings Asian salad (page 26)

serves 6

Preheat the oven to 160°C (325°F, Gas Mark 2). Heat the olive oil in a large frying pan and sauté the onions, garlic and herbs until the onion is very soft. Peel the kumara, chop roughly, then boil for 20 minutes or until soft. Drain, then puree in a food processor with the apple concentrate, corn oil and tofu until completely smooth. Season with salt and pepper. Peel and core the apple and slice finely. Spread the onion mixture over the base of the pastry shell, lay the apple slices on top, then finish with the kumara mash. Sprinkle with the nigella seeds and bake for 25 minutes. Serve with the Asian salad.

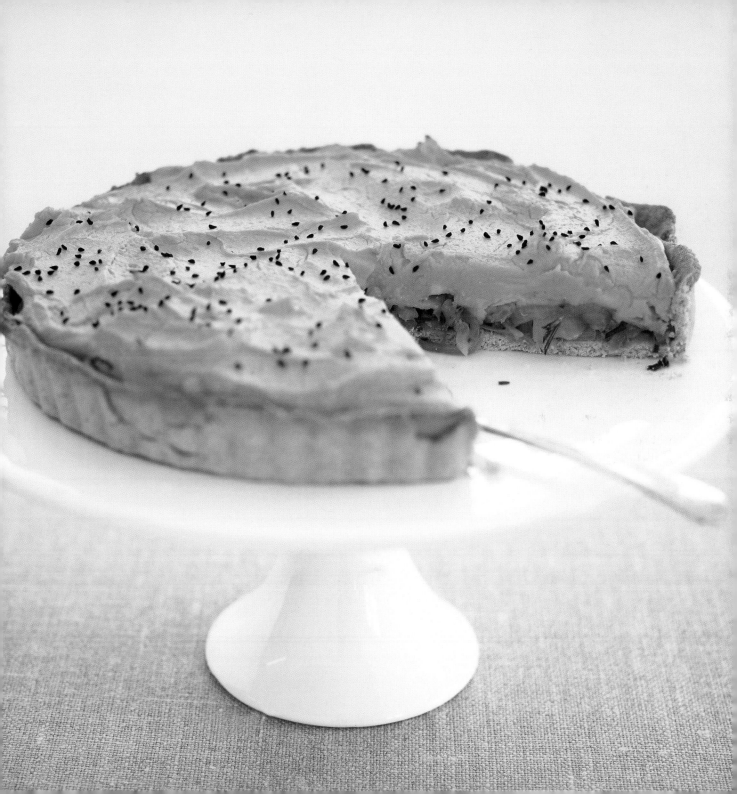

It seems hypocritical to happily munch fish but not eat meat for moral reasons, yet I do! The prospect of going to the fish markets fills me with excitement, so much so that I even take tourists there, believing it will be as exciting for them as their first glimpse of the Opera House. The health benefits of fish are so great that I will not allow myself to become consumed by moral conflict over eating it. With the busy lives we lead it's hard to fulfil our body's protein requirements without eating meat and seafood. It's possible, but it takes much more time and planning.

In Scotland we ate fish and chips – luckily not too often, as my mother was frightened of the chip pan – kippers and Arbroath smokies (smoked haddock), lemon sole in white sauce and fish pie (fish in a creamy white sauce with potatoes). It was bland in colour and most unexciting. There is a fish restaurant in Darlinghurst, Sydney, that taught me to think outside that 'Scottish square' and combine fish with a variety of things. All you need to do is understand the flavours – delicate fish can't be overwhelmed.

The great thing about fish is that it is quick to cook, easy to digest and full of wonderful oils that the body responds to so well. For those who believe they can't cook fish and reserve the pleasure of eating it for going out, there are a few tricks that I hope will help.

seafood

baked ocean trout with bean mash and asian greens

❝Men like mash. It's true, and no matter how many times I try to convince them that it is better to restrict their intake of starchy foods like potato, bread, pasta and rice at night, many feel dissatisfied without a hearty carb on their plate. Many men also dislike legumes, or so they think . . . Enter the world of mashed legumes. Disguise legumes with different flavours, and men (and children) will be scoffing them down and licking their plates, with absolutely no idea of what they've just eaten. This mash can be made in advance and heated just before serving. ❞

4 x 125 g (4 oz) ocean trout fillets

juice of 1 lime

½ bunch fresh coriander (cilantro),
   chopped

4 servings stir-fried Asian greens
   (page 28)

mash

2½ cups cooked (or canned) haricot
   (navy) beans (see page 177–8)

1 tablespoon water, reserved from
   cooking the beans (or from the can)

1 clove garlic, crushed

1 tablespoon chopped fresh dill

2 tablespoons miso dressing
   (page 15)

serves 4

To make the bean mash, blend the beans, reserved water, garlic and dill together in a food processor. Slowly add the miso dressing until the mixture is completely smooth but not too runny (you may have dressing left over). Set the mash aside ready to be heated just before serving.

Preheat the oven to 180°C (350°F, Gas Mark 4). Make four individual foil parcels and place one trout fillet in each. Drizzle with the lime juice, sprinkle over the coriander and seal each parcel loosely. Bake for 15–20 minutes.

Heat the mash in a pan or in the microwave and serve with the fish and the stir-fried Asian greens.

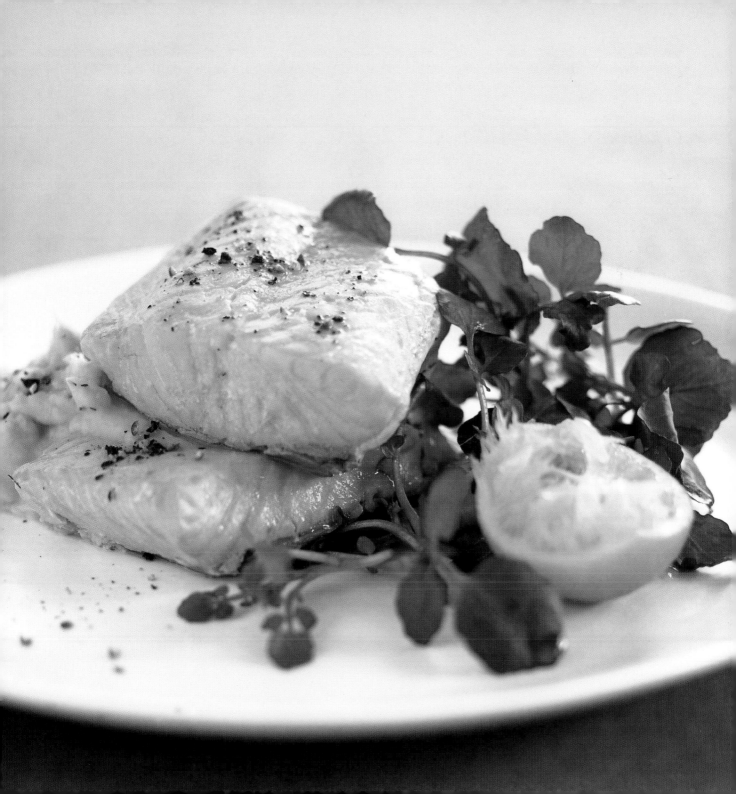

blue-eye cod with papaya and beansprout salsa

" Papaya for summer. Beansprouts for vitality. Add to them the wonderful healthy properties of fish, and this dish will make you feel ready to **take on the world. ""**

4 x 125 g (4 oz) fillets blue-eye cod

juice of 1 lime

1 tablespoon chilli oil

1–2 tablespoons chopped fresh
   coriander (cilantro)

4 sprigs fresh coriander (cilantro), to serve

4 servings stir-fried Asian greens
   (page 28)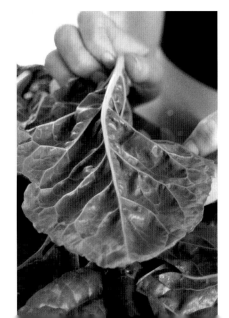

salsa

2 cups thinly sliced red papaya (pawpaw)

3 cups beansprouts

1 cup grated Lebanese cucumber

1 green chilli, seeded and finely chopped

2 tablespoons finely chopped fresh mint

1 cup fresh roughly chopped
   coriander (cilantro)

pinch sea salt

cracked black pepper, to taste

juice of 2 limes

serves 4

Preheat the oven to 180°C (350°F, Gas Mark 4). Wipe the fillets with a damp paper towel and pat dry. Squeeze a third of the lime juice over the fillets then, using a pastry brush, lightly brush chilli oil over one side of each fillet. Top each fillet with a pinch of chopped coriander before loosely wrapping each in its own sealed foil parcel.

To make the salsa, combine the papaya, beansprouts, cucumber, chilli, mint and coriander in a bowl. Season with salt and pepper and pour over the lime juice. Refrigerate for at least 1 hour before serving.

Bake the fish parcels on a baking tray for 15 minutes. Serve the fish on a bed of salsa with a sprig of coriander on top and stir-fried Asian greens on the side.

grilled tuna and beans with chilli-limed hummus and slow-roasted tomatoes

"During a week's stay at the home of my good friends Mark and Robert in Byron Bay, I was instructed to coach them. A pantry and fridge audit uncovered **ghosts of dinner parties very much past**. I boxed up their snack foods so that they were still on hand 'in case guests dropped in', and the boys responded well . . . until guests *did* drop in – eleven of them! The box was ripped open and out came the cheese, crackers, chips and chocolates. The boys were in an entertainers' frenzy that was near impossible to contain. The main meal was mine, though (with conditions attached). The tuna had to have 'height', colour and flavour, and if I could achieve all these things and make it healthy as well, even better.

This meal achieves all those demands and, best of all, it can be prepared in advance before the guests arrive. It's simply a matter of steaming the beans, grilling the tuna and piecing it all together. Chilli oils vary according to brand – check for strength and adjust the quantity according to taste. "

6 x 125 g (4 oz) tuna steaks

juice of 3 limes

¼ cup olive oil

1 clove garlic, chopped

1 cup chopped fresh coriander
  (cilantro)

pinch sea salt

cracked black pepper, to taste

1 kg (2 lb) yellow and green beans
  ends trimmed >

Prepare the tomatoes first (see over). While they are roasting, place the tuna steaks in a dish and cover with the combined lime juice, olive oil, garlic, coriander and seasoning. Cover in plastic wrap and refrigerate for at least 1 hour.

Wash and top and tail the beans and place them in a steamer. Heat the grill to hot and put the beans on to steam. Ensure that your barbecue or chargrill pan is well oiled so your tuna won't stick. Grill the tuna steaks for 2–3 minutes on each side, turning once only. Remove the beans from the heat. >

tomatoes

9 Roma (plum) tomatoes, halved

1 tablespoon olive oil

1 teaspoon chilli oil

hummus

1 quantity hummus (page 18), made
  using lime rather than lemon juice

2 tablespoons olive oil

1 teaspoon chilli oil

serves 6

To prepare the tomatoes, preheat the oven to 120°C (250°F, Gas Mark 1) and brush each tomato half with a mix of the two oils. Place in the oven and roast slowly for approximately 3 hours. The tomatoes will happily keep warm for longer if needed; just turn the oven down to 50°C (100°F).

Put some hummus on each plate, mix together the olive oil and chilli oil and drizzle a little over the hummus. Place three tomato halves on each plate, the beans on top of the hummus and the tuna on top of the beans.

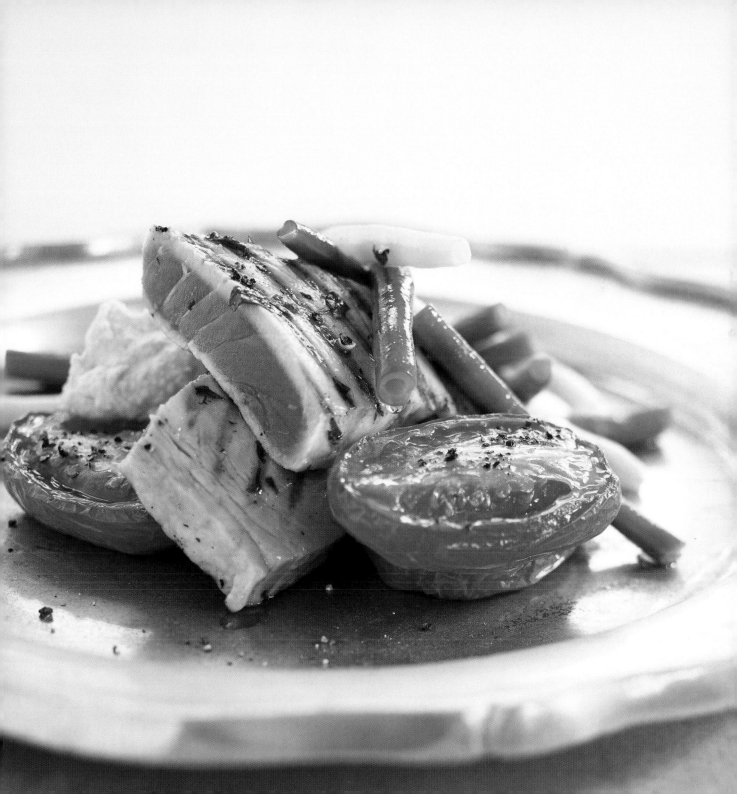

calamari and lime salad

"It's all about summer, this dish. If you think in pictures, then imagine that the outside table is laid. It's a lovely warm day and you're looking forward to friends coming over. What could make a nicer **lunch on a hot summer day** than this salad, served with warmed wholegrain sourdough bread? Or serve it as a starter on a summer evening, before the boys get the barbeque going. You can substitute whitebait for the calamari if you prefer."

1 tablespoon olive oil

350 g (11 oz) calamari rings

½ red chilli, seeded and finely
   chopped

juice of 1 lime

2–4 servings Asian salad (page 26;
   keep the dressing separate until
   ready to serve)

1 avocado, sliced

1 red capsicum (bell pepper), cut into
   thin strips

3 spring onions (scallions), cut
   lengthways into thin slices about
   5 cm (2 in) long

serves 4 as a starter or 2 as a main

Heat the olive oil in a wok over a high heat and quickly stir-fry the calamari rings and the chilli until the calamari is opaque and tender. Transfer to a bowl and squeeze over the lime juice. Arrange some of the Asian salad on each plate, decorate with the avocado, capsicum and spring onions, put the calamari on top and drizzle with Asian salad dressing.

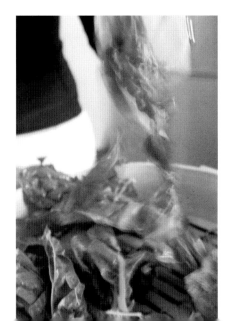

baked mackerel

"I developed a taste for mackerel on holiday with my sister, Jennifer, and my cousins, Fiona and Duncan. We stayed in a pretty little town in the north-west of Scotland called Kinlochbervie. Duncan and I preferred fishing to sightseeing or picnicking with our elder sisters, so we would head off to the pier and happily spend the day fishing for mackerel. The fish appeared to jump onto any line with a shiny hook, so we caught plenty. Our sisters told us with great amusement that the locals believed mackerel to be dirty and only of use as bait. Whether Duncan and I liked mackerel or not, in defiance of our sisters we carried our catch home each night and ate the spoils of our labour, carefully prepared by my Auntie Irene. Thirty years later, I'm not too mature to dismiss the opportunity to seek retribution for many days of teasing – this recipe is for Jennifer and Fiona. Mackerel is delicious, easy to prepare and relatively inexpensive. It's also an extremely good source of nutrients. Steer clear of the very large fish, as an extra precaution against ingestion of mercury."

2 tablespoons pine nuts

1 bunch watercress

1 tablespoon preserved lemon
(page 16)

1 tablespoon olive oil

2.5 kg (5 lb) mackerel, cleaned

serves 6

Preheat the oven to 180°C (350°F, Gas Mark 4). Roast the pine nuts in dry pan until golden and set aside. Remove and discard the thicker stalks from the watercress, then puree in a blender, adding the pine nuts and preserved lemon and finally pouring the olive oil into the mix. Make sure the fish is completely clean, and wipe over with paper towel or a dry tea towel. Score the skin of the fish and smear the watercress paste all over the fish, inside and out. Wrap the fish in foil, place on a baking tray and bake in the oven for 30 minutes before removing the foil and baking for a further 15 minutes. This tastes great served with grilled mushrooms drizzled with a dressing of shoyu (soy sauce) and lemon juice, and steamed Asian greens.

baked snapper

"It took me some time to take on a whole fish, but once I did I couldn't work out why I had resisted for so long. Ask your fishmonger (nicely) to clean and scale the fish thoroughly. They might also be persuaded to trim the gills and other sharp, protruding bits. Make sure it is thoroughly scaled; the meal can be ruined if you get a mouthful of fish scales. Wash the fish thoroughly inside and out and pat it dry with paper towel or a clean tea towel. It might also be nice if you **thanked it very sincerely** for giving up its life for you. "

2 tablespoons slivered almonds

1 cup finely chopped fresh flat-leaf parsley

1 tablespoon chopped preserved lemon (page 16) or the juice of 1 large lemon

⅓ cup olive oil

1.5 kg (3 lb) whole snapper, cleaned

1 large clove garlic, cut into fine slivers

serves 4

Preheat the oven to 180°C (350°F, Gas Mark 4). In a dry pan, roast the almonds over a medium heat until they give off a delicious toasty aroma. Mix the parsley with the preserved lemon or lemon juice, then slowly pour in the olive oil while stirring to make a paste. Score the outside of the fish about 1 cm (½ in) deep a few times and stab garlic into the gashes. Smear the paste all over the inside and outside of the fish, pressing the mixture firmly into the outside cuts. Sprinkle the almonds into the cavity of the fish. Wrap the fish in foil and bake for 20 minutes. Remove the foil and continue to bake for a further 10–15 minutes until the skin is crunchy. This is delicious served with fatoush (page 32) and kumara chips (page 66).

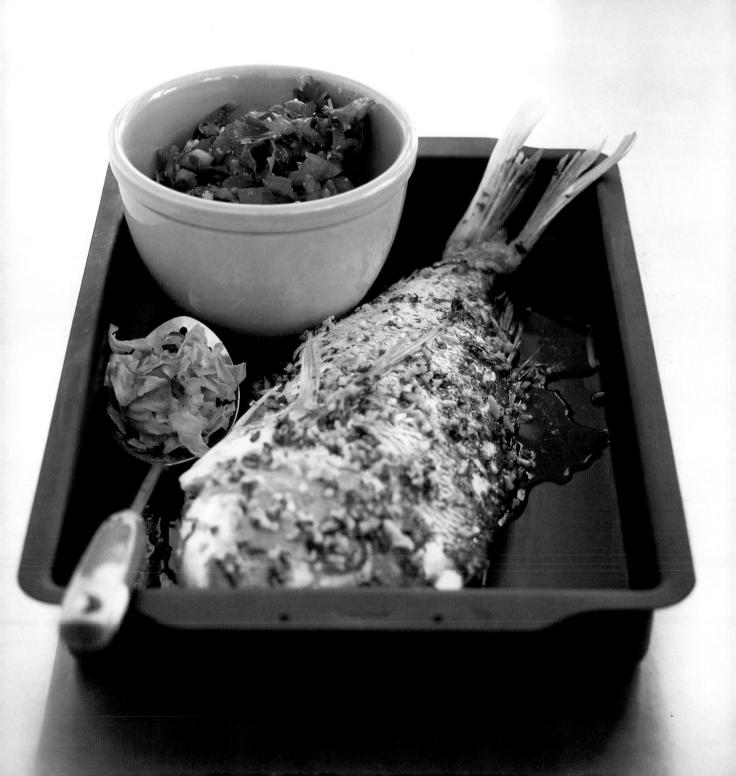

baked asian salmon

"It's a bit of a rort this recipe: Blind Freddy (whoever he was) could see that there is no great skill involved and I couldn't possibly lay exclusive claim to writing it. Who could? It's in here because 'gate to plate' there is nothing easier and, during the week, when you are tired and tempted to get takeaway, this is a good one to pull out of the hat. You're through the gate and in the door. Turn on the oven to heat up and take the salmon out of the fridge. From there it's just a quick chop, squeeze and wrap before you've got the fish in the oven, you're up the stairs changing your clothes and 15 minutes later it's ready. Don't forget the greens. For health and speed nothing beats this meal. "

1 tablespoon mirin

½ tablespoon shoyu (soy sauce)

¼ cup chopped fresh coriander
   (cilantro)

juice of ½ lime

2 x 125 g (4 oz) fillets salmon

2 servings stir-fried Asian greens
   (page 28)

serves 2

Preheat the oven to 180°C (350°F, Gas Mark 4). Mix the mirin, shoyu, coriander and lime juice together in a bowl. Wipe the fish with damp paper towel and lay each fillet on a sheet of foil. Lift the edges of the foil up around each fillet to make four walls before spooning the mirin mixture over each one. Wrap the foil around the fish in a loose parcel and bake for 15 minutes. Serve with the stir-fried Asian greens.

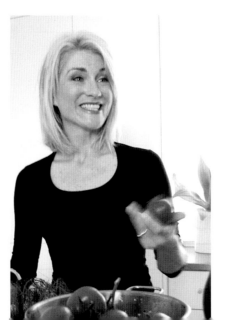

beetroot and sun-dried tomato salsa with blue-eye cod and green lentils

" Food coaching men can be difficult, as most don't feel satisfied unless their plate is stacked with potatoes or chips. The game, therefore, is to encourage them to improve their health without them feeling they have sacrificed too much. I tested this recipe on one of the 'bloke-iest' of my clients, who eyed the plate suspiciously at first. The lentils quite obviously set alarm bells ringing, as he picked up his cutlery with trepidation. His eating pace accelerated with each mouthful and the clean plate suggested that the meal was not that bad. If you are trying to **steer away from chips**, potatoes, pasta and rice to more healthful mashed legumes and lentils, don't forget the kombu when cooking the lentils – it helps prevent flatulence! The salsa is also delicious served on its own with crudités or flat bread, or as a filling for tartlets (see page 59). "

salsa

1 cup sun-dried tomatoes

1 clove garlic, crushed

1 small red chilli, seeded and finely
  chopped

4 tablespoons olive oil

2 medium-sized roast beetroot (beet)
  (page 23)

juice of 1 lemon

cracked black pepper, to taste >

To make the salsa, blend the tomatoes, garlic, chilli and oil in a food processor until the tomatoes are quite finely chopped. Add the beetroot and lemon juice and continue to process until the mixture is fine but still quite textured in consistency. Season with pepper. If required, add a little water (1 tablespoon) to the mixture, to make the salsa a little smoother. >

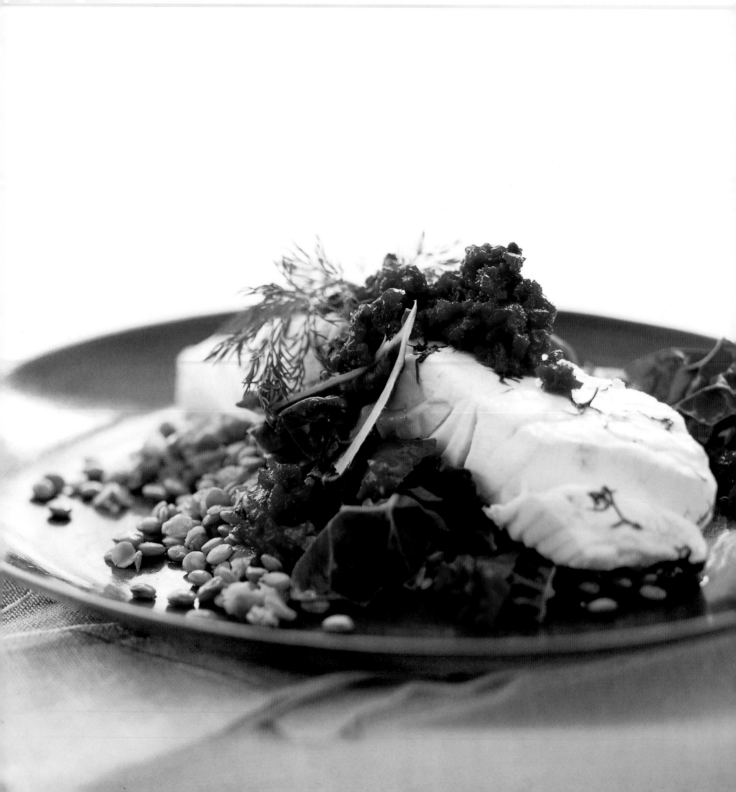

1½ cups Australian green or Puy lentils

5 cups water

1 x 10 cm (4 in) strip kombu

1 carrot, peeled and very roughly
  chopped

1 stick celery

1 bay leaf

1 small onion, peeled and quartered

pinch sea salt

few sprigs fresh dill

6 x 125 g (4 oz) blue-eye cod fillets

serves 6

To prepare the lentils, rinse in cold water before putting in a pan with the 5 cups of water and kombu. Add the carrot, celery, bay leaf and onion and bring to the boil. As soon as the water has boiled, remove and discard the kombu. Reduce the heat and simmer the lentils for 20–25 minutes or until tender, adding the salt in the last 5 minutes of cooking.

While the lentils are cooking, choose a pan wide enough to fit the fish fillets in a single layer. Put in enough water to cover the fish, add the dill sprigs and bring the water to the boil. Reduce the heat and poach the fillets for 8–15 minutes – the cooking time will vary depending on the fillets. To check whether the fish is cooked, gently pierce the flesh with a knife – it should be opaque. Once the fish is cooked, drain the lentils and discard the carrots, onion, bay leaf and celery. Serve the fish on a bed of lentils and top with the salsa.

chargrilled ocean perch and kumara mash

" Nothing very complicated with this one. It's another 'gate to plate' dish that takes just minutes. If you have a decent fish shop en route from work, grab a couple of pieces of fresh ocean perch and you'll have a delicious meal on your plate in minutes. Perch is such a lovely light, clean-tasting fish and complements the flavours of za'tar beautifully. "

1 medium-sized kumara (sweet potato), peeled and chopped into 2.5 cm (1 in) pieces

2 x 125 g (4 oz) ocean perch fillets

2 tablespoons za'tar (page 15)

1 tablespoon olive oil

1 bunch English spinach

serves 2

Steam the kumara for 20 minutes or until tender, then mash. While the kumara is steaming, preheat the grill (broiler) to hot, wipe the perch fillets with damp paper towel and pat dry. In a small bowl mix the za'tar with enough of the olive oil to make a paste. Using a flat knife, smear the za'tar paste over each side of the fish. Grill (broil) for 3 minutes on each side. Meanwhile, steam the English spinach for 3 minutes or until wilted. Serve the perch on the mashed kumara with steamed English spinach on the side.

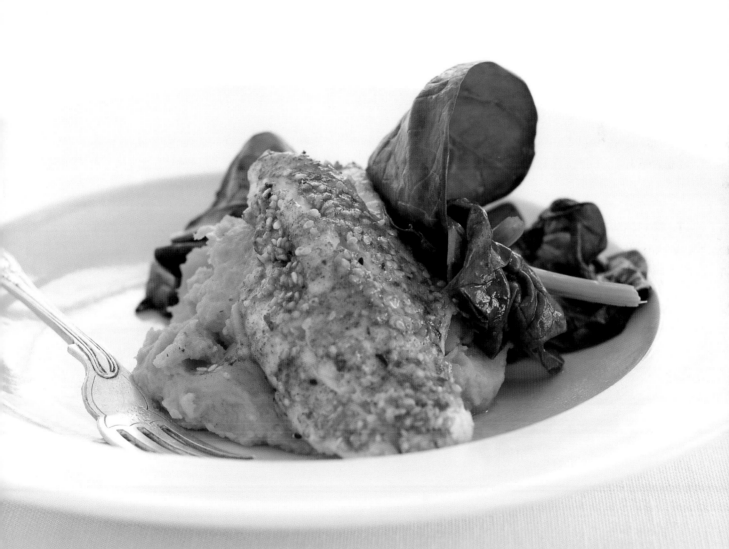

redfish fishcakes with chilli jam

"My goddaughter, Laura, recently asked me why I was always talking about food. She did have a point. If I'm not talking about food, I'm thinking about it. **I even dream of meals** that I ate years ago, remembering how delicious they were. One meal I remember eating nine years ago was fishcakes with chilli jam, and I'd like to share with you my interpretation of the same meal. This recipe for fishcakes was adapted from one from the Sydney Fish Market. I've changed some of the ingredients so the flavours work better with the chilli jam and to make it a little healthier. Use a non-stick frying pan so you can reduce the amount of oil required for shallow-frying. You can buy chilli jam from a good deli if you decide not to make your own."

chilli jam

1 tablespoon olive oil

500 g (1 lb) ripe tomatoes, halved

2 teaspoons cumin seeds

2 teaspoons mustard seeds

3 cloves garlic, crushed

2 fresh red chillies, seeded and finely chopped

2.5 cm (1 in) knob fresh ginger, grated

¼ cup red wine vinegar

¼ cup rice syrup

1 tablespoon fish sauce >

To make the chilli jam, preheat the oven to 180°C (350°F, Gas Mark 4), pour the olive oil into a roasting tray, add the tomatoes and roast for 20 minutes. Dry-roast the cumin and mustard seeds in a frying pan and, once fragrant, remove and crush with a mortar and pestle. In a heavy-based pan, combine the spices with the garlic, chilli, ginger, vinegar, rice syrup and fish sauce and heat gently. Add the tomatoes to the saucepan and simmer for 1½ hours, stirring occasionally, until the mixture thickens and looks like jam. Pour into a sterilised jar and seal while hot. >

fishcakes

500 g (1 lb) redfish (red drum) fillets

zest of 1 lemon

1 teaspoon fish sauce

½ bunch spring onions (scallions),
   chopped

½ teaspoon sea salt

cracked black pepper, to taste

3 medium-sized desiree potatoes

5 teaspoons olive oil

½ cup finely shredded rocket (arugula)

4 servings Italian green salad
   (page 27)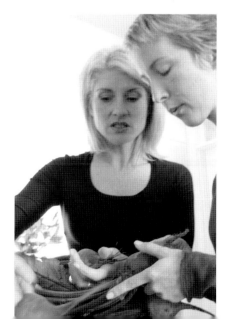

makes 8 fishcakes and 1 cup chilli jam

While the chilli jam is simmering, make the fishcakes. Using a damp, clean cloth, wipe the redfish clean and ensure it is free of scales and skin. Place the fish, lemon zest, fish sauce, spring onions and seasoning in a food processor and process until the fish is finely minced (ground). Peel and cut the potatoes into chunks and steam until cooked through. Mash in a bowl with 1 teaspoon of the olive oil. Add the fish mixture to the potatoes and fold through the rocket until well combined. With wet hands, mould into eight patties, each about 10 cm (4 in) in diameter, and refrigerate until ready to cook. In a large non-stick frying pan, heat the remaining olive oil and shallow-fry the patties for 4 minutes each side, turning once. Serve the fishcakes with the chilli jam and Italian green salad.

moonfish with cucumber and lemon salsa

" I first had moonfish at a restaurant in North Sydney. It was served with a parmesan, pine nut and herb crust on a bed of pickled cucumber. The **flavour and texture** of the fish was delightful. Moonfish is perfect for people who are put off fish by the smell and the bones, as it is large, fleshy and quite odourless. If you can't find moonfish, use deep-sea ocean perch, swordfish or ling and select the thickest fillets. "

½ cup pine nuts

2 tablespoons chopped fresh
    rosemary

4 x 125 g (4 oz) pieces moonfish
    (opah), skinned

slivers preserved lemon (page 16),
    to serve

beetroot greens (page 24) or steamed
    English spinach, to serve

salsa

2 Lebanese cucumbers, peeled

2 x 2.5 cm (1 in) pieces preserved
    lemon (page 16), finely chopped

1 tablespoon chopped fresh mint

juice of 1 lemon

serves 4

To make the salsa, use a vegetable peeler to slice the cucumbers thinly length-ways. Place the slices in a bowl and add the preserved lemon, mint and lemon juice. Mix it all together and rest a plate on the surface to weigh the ingredients down. Chill in the fridge for 2–3 hours.

Grind the pine nuts and rosemary together in a spice grinder. Press the mixture over each side of the moonfish with the blade of a knife. Cover the barbecue or chargrill plate with foil and grill the fish over a moderate heat for 4 minutes on each side, taking care not to burn the pine nuts in the crust. Place a few slivers of preserved lemon on top of the fish and serve it with the cucumber and lemon salsa and steamed greens.

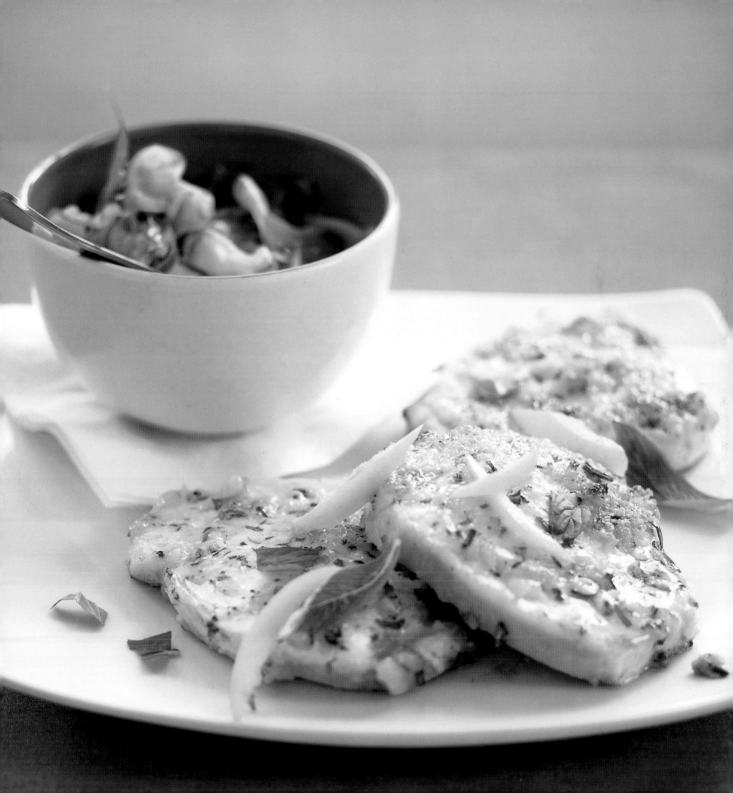

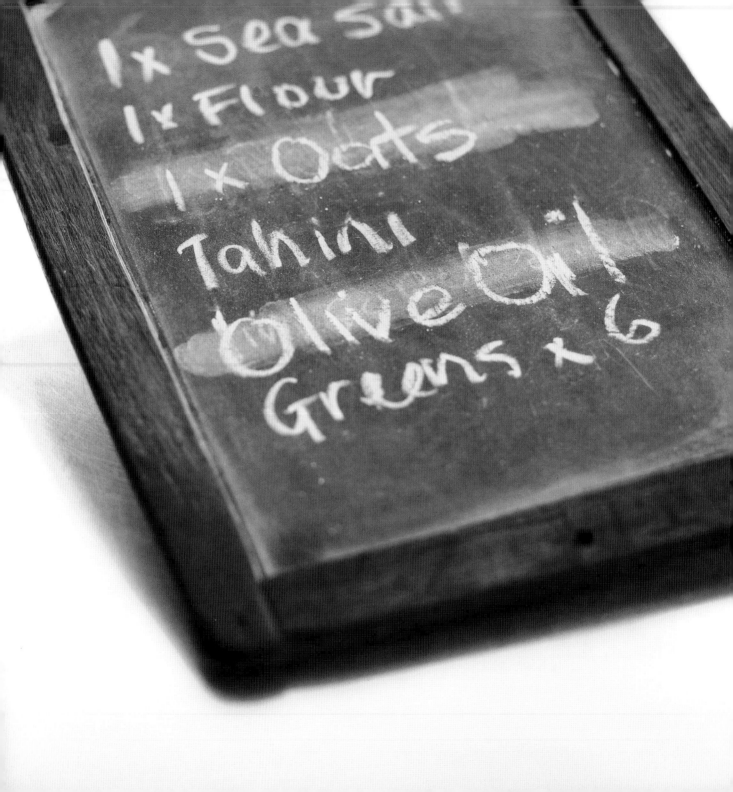

1x Sea Salt
1x Flour
1x Oats
Tahini
Olive Oil
Greens x 6

grilled tuna and roast almond pesto

" This meal is quite **delicious and very substantial**. Select small tuna steaks for this dish, as it is quite rich. "

4 x 125 g (4 oz) tuna steaks

2 tablespoons olive oil

juice of 1 lemon

sea salt, to taste

cracked black pepper, to taste

4 servings seasoned spinach and
   olive oil (page 27)

pesto

½ cup raw almonds

1 clove garlic

juice of 1 lemon

½ cup fresh flat-leaf parsley

½ cup rocket (arugula) leaves

½ cup light olive oil

1 tablespoon capers, rinsed
   and drained

serves 4

Wipe both sides of the tuna steaks with damp paper towel. Mix the olive oil, lemon juice and seasoning together and drizzle over the fish, turning each steak to ensure that both sides are coated with the marinade. Set aside while you make the pesto.

To make the pesto, dry-roast the almonds over a medium heat for 5 minutes or until they darken. Set aside to cool then mix with the other pesto ingredients in a food processor until well combined but still quite grainy. Refrigerate until ready to serve.

Heat a well-seasoned chargrill pan or barbecue and cook the tuna steaks for 3–5 minutes on each side, turning them once. Serve on a bed of spinach and top with the pesto sauce.

clams and garlic polenta

"I recently accepted a challenge from the marketing manager of the Sydney Fish Market to cook with a new species of fish each week. The Sydney Fish Market is the second largest in the world after Tokyo. With so many different types of fish, I suspect I'll regret the challenge in five years' time, but I'm sure my body won't.

Clams, or vongole, are simple to prepare, very tasty and easy to eat. Due to their size, I find them less overwhelming to eat than mussels. This dish is very easy, particularly if you already have a batch of Dina's tomato sauce in the freezer or fridge. It could be served with pasta, but this garlic polenta is a nice alternative; the yellow of the polenta contrasts so beautifully with the red of the tomato sauce. This recipe is also great for those who are **intolerant of wheat products** and can't eat bread or pasta."

1 kg (2 lb) clams (vongole)

9 cups water

1 x 10 cm (4 in) piece kombu

½ teaspoon sea salt

1½ cups polenta (cornmeal)

3 cloves garlic, crushed

2 tablespoons olive oil

2 cups Dina's tomato sauce
(page 20)

4 servings Italian green salad
(page 27)

serves 4

To avoid a mouthful of grit, molluscs like clams should be purged. To do this, simply put them in a large bowl of cool water and leave for 30–40 minutes. Once purged, give them a rinse and they are ready to cook.

Put the water and kombu in a large pan and bring to the boil. Remove the kombu and add the salt and polenta, stirring continuously. When the polenta starts to splutter, turn the heat to low and simmer, stirring occasionally, for 40 minutes or until cooked (polenta is cooked when it pulls away from the sides of the pan). Remove from the heat, spread thinly over a flat baking sheet and leave to cool. Mix the garlic with the olive oil in a bowl and heat the grill (broiler) to hot. Once the polenta is cool, cut into eight squares and brush the surface of each with the garlic oil. Place under the hot grill (broiler) for 10 minutes, until it starts to become crispy and golden. Turn and cook the other side until golden.

Heat the tomato sauce in a large pan and, once hot, add the clams, stirring them through the sauce. Cover and cook over a high heat for 6 minutes or until the clams have opened. Serve with the polenta and Italian green salad.

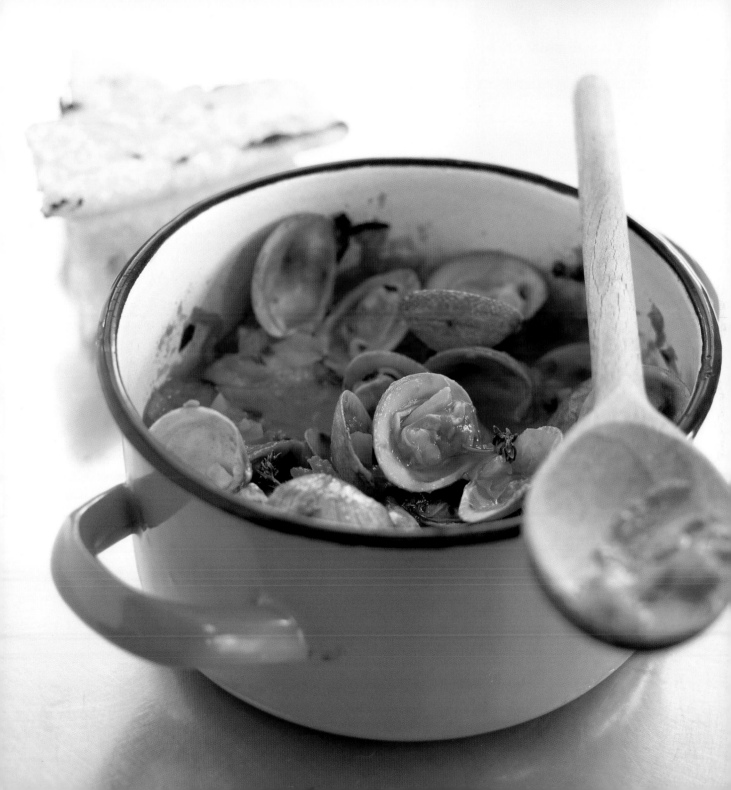

When clients come to me expressing a wish to lose weight, I encourage them to stick to dinners of a serve of lean protein with vegetables (mainly greens, of course) and no bread, rice or pasta. Chicken, lean meat, seafood and tofu are the best sources of protein. Eggs and cheese are high in cholesterol and should be eaten in moderation.

Vegetarians who don't plan their diet carefully tend to eat meals that are high in fat and carbohydrates. A diet of bread, rice, pasta, cheese with a few vegetables can cause many to put on weight, particularly those who are less active and past their mid-twenties.

For better health I encourage you to buy organic meat (especially chicken) and to restrict your consumption of red meat to no more than twice a week. Because I choose not to eat meat, there are only a few meat meals in this book, but I am assured that they are good. I recommend them if you are trying to cajole a diehard 'doesn't like health food' person into eating more healthily.

chicken
& red meat

lemon za'tar chicken with chargrilled zucchini and spinach

❝ When my friend Melinda said that she was testing this recipe on her in-laws I was unsure whether she liked the sound of the dish or just wanted a good excuse to inflict something terrible on them for dinner. By all accounts they loved it, and Melinda was elevated to great heights that night for serving such a scrumptious meal. This is a great dish for people who are **trying to lose weight** – served with simple steamed greens, the za'tar gives life to the meal. ❞

4 organic corn-fed chicken breast
   fillets

1 egg white, lightly beaten

4 tablespoons za'tar (page 15)

4 zucchinis (courgettes)

2 tablespoons olive oil

sea salt, to taste

1 lemon, cut into 3 mm (⅛ in) slices

1 bunch English spinach

serves 4

Lightly score the chicken fillets before dipping them in the egg white and coating with the za'tar.

Wash the zucchinis, cut lengthways into strips about 5 mm (¼ in) thick, brush each strip with olive oil and sprinkle with sea salt.

Heat a well-oiled barbecue or chargrill pan and grill the chicken fillets for 6–8 minutes each side, depending on their thickness. Add the zucchini strips 5 minutes after you put the chicken on to cook, and grill for about 3 minutes each side. Add the lemon slices in the last 2 minutes.

Steam the spinach for 2 minutes and drain well. Serve the chicken with the zucchini and lemon slices on top and the spinach on the side.

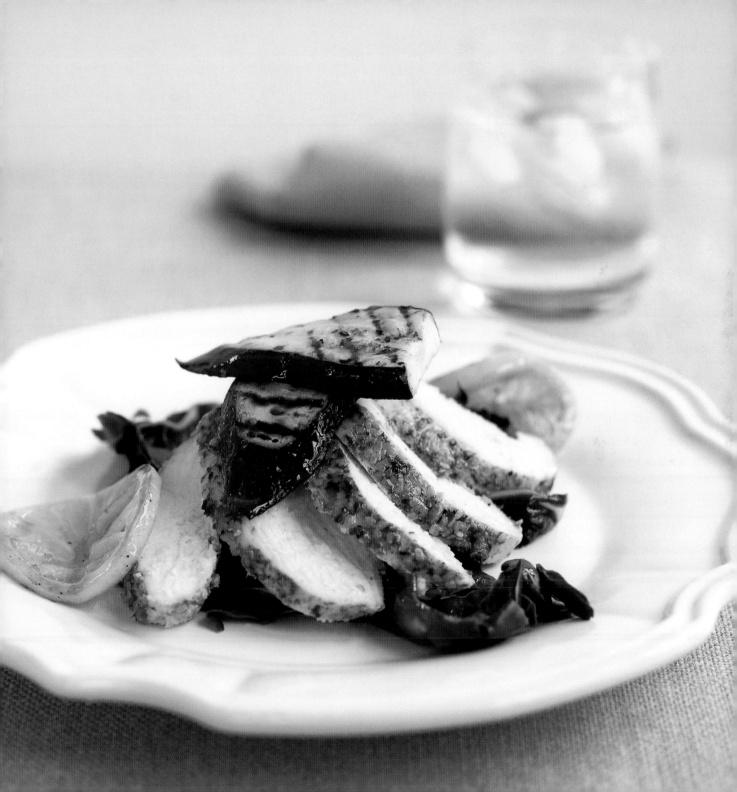

beefburgers with tomato and bean salsa

" This one is for Su, my first client and possibly my greatest challenge. Su exposed me to eating habits worse than I could ever have imagined – a world of takeaway food, chips, chicken salt and packaged foods. My world of legumes, greens and whole grains was every bit as unfamiliar to her. Bit by bit, each of us made compromises until we arrived at common ground.

If you love takeaway burgers, the shift to vegetable patties and mung beans is possibly a bit radical (although I did try in the early days!), so for Su, and burger-lovers everywhere, this recipe is slipped in to entice you away from the processed, mass-produced stuff and towards **a preference for real food**. Most beefburgers are made using fatty meat, which makes them moist. Using rump steak with all the fat trimmed off will make this version a little drier, but with the delicious bean and tomato salsa you will never know the difference. These are just as tasty and, of course, much better for you. Don't use salt to season the meat, as it will draw moisture from it. "

salsa

1 tablespoon olive oil

1 small brown onion, finely chopped

1 small red chilli, seeded and finely
  chopped

3 cloves garlic, crushed

1 teaspoon ground cumin

½ teaspoon sweet paprika

2 x 400 g (13 oz) cans Roma (plum)
  tomatoes

1 x 400 g (13 oz) can organic kidney
  beans >

To make the salsa, heat the oil in a medium saucepan and sauté the onion and chilli until the onion is soft. Add the garlic, cumin and paprika and sauté for a further 2 minutes. Break the tomatoes into small chunks in a bowl before adding them to the pan. Bring the tomato mixture to the boil then reduce the heat and simmer for 30 minutes. Drain the kidney beans and add to the salsa. Return to the boil, reduce heat and simmer for a further 20 minutes. >

burgers

500 g (1 lb) rump steak

½ onion, finely chopped

½ cup fresh flat-leaf parsley,
   finely chopped

freshly ground black pepper, to taste

1 tablespoon olive oil

4 servings Italian green salad
   (page 27)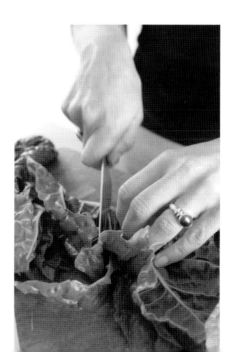

serves 4

Preheat a barbecue or well-seasoned chargrill pan to hot. Trim the fat off the steak and chop in a food processor until it looks like minced (ground) beef. Add the onion, parsley and pepper and mix through. Divide the mixture into 4 patties and press them firmly into shape. Brush each patty with a little oil and cook for 3–6 minutes on each side, turning once. Spoon the salsa over the patties and serve with the Italian green salad.

moroccan lamb with fennel and olives

" I'm a huge fan of fennel. Serve it with red meat and it will help **facilitate complete digestion**. This meal is super-easy and makes a good mid-week dinner party dish. Once the fennel and dressing are prepared, just stick the vegetables in the oven, heat the grill and cook the lamb – and thirty minutes later you'll be sitting down to a meal your guests will love. "

1 tablespoon cumin seeds

1 teaspoon fresh thyme leaves

¼ cup finely chopped fresh mint

juice of 1 lemon

½ teaspoon honey

½ cup olive oil

500 g (1 lb) trim lamb fillets

   (or 12 cutlets with fat trimmed off)

3 bulbs fennel (finocchio)

1 tablespoon olive oil

½ cup kalamata olives, seeded and

   halved

4 servings seasoned spinach and

   olive oil (page 27)

serves 4

Dry-roast the cumin seeds then grind to a fine powder using a mortar and pestle or spice grinder. Combine the cumin with the thyme, mint, lemon, honey and the ½ cup of olive oil to make a thick dressing. Put the lamb in a bowl, pour over half the dressing and leave to marinate at room temperature for about 1 hour. Reserve the rest of the dressing.

Preheat the oven to 160°C (325°F, Gas Mark 3) and heat the grill (broiler) or barbecue to hot. Prepare the fennel by trimming the top off the bulbs, removing the wispy leaves and outer layers, and cutting off the hard bottom core. Cut each bulb diagonally into 6 pieces. Bring a large pan of salted water to the boil and add the fennel. When the water comes to the boil again, remove from the heat and drain the fennel. Heat the tablespoon of olive oil in a roasting tin and add the fennel and the olives. Roast for 15 minutes, turning occasionally. While the fennel is roasting, grill (broil) or barbecue the lamb for 10–15 minutes, turning once only. Remove the fennel from the oven and stir through the remainder of the dressing. Serve with the lamb on top and spinach on the side.

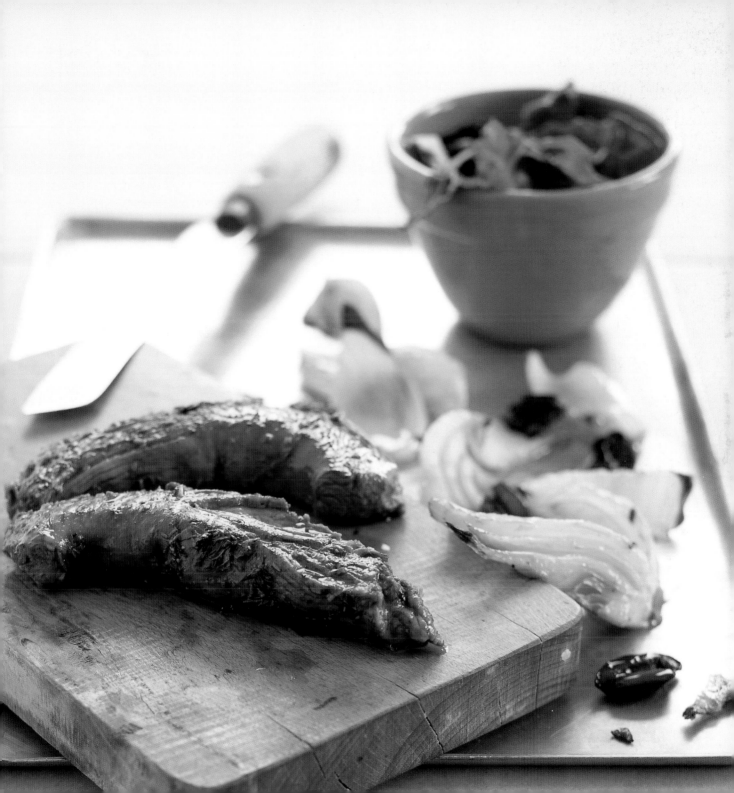

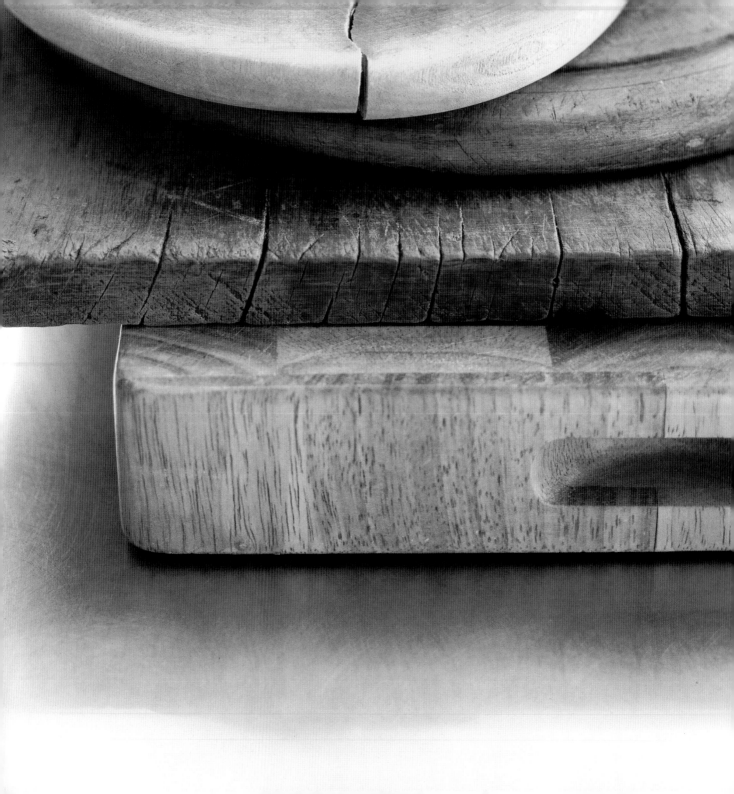

chicken kebabs

" My good friend Melinda is married to **a dedicated carnivore** who takes great delight in ribbing me continually about 'horrible health food'. One of Greg's favourite breakfasts is a packet of crisps in a bread roll – need I go on? With great fear and trepidation I gave Melinda my entire collection of meat dishes to test and rate – meeting Greg's approval was the ultimate challenge. While they didn't all pass his stringent criteria, most did, and these kebabs were one of his favourites. **""**

1 large clove garlic, crushed

1 red chilli, seeded and finely chopped

1 x 2.5 cm (1 in) knob ginger, grated

juice of 1 lime or lemon

½ cup chopped mixed herbs, such
   as lemongrass, mint, coriander
   (cilantro) and parsley

⅓ cup olive oil

1 teaspoon fish sauce

350 g (11 oz) chicken breast fillet

1 large red capsicum (bell pepper)

1 large Spanish (red) onion

24 button mushrooms or 12 larger
   mushrooms, cleaned, stalks
   removed

8 bamboo skewers, soaked in water
   for about 10 minutes

4 servings stir-fried Asian greens
   (page 28)

serves 4

Heat the grill (broiler) or barbecue to hot. Mix together the garlic, chilli, ginger, lime or lemon juice, herbs, oil and fish sauce. Cut the chicken, capsicum and onion into 2.5 cm (1 in) chunks and halve or quarter the mushrooms. Put the chicken, capsicum, onion and mushroom pieces in a bowl and pour over the marinade, mixing thoroughly to ensure all the pieces are coated. Marinate overnight or for at least 4 hours before threading the meat and vegetables onto the bamboo skewers.

Pour any remaining marinade over the kebabs and grill (broil) or barbecue them, turning occasionally, for 10 minutes or until the chicken is cooked through. Serve with the stir-fried Asian greens.

fillet steak with caper and olive salsa

" I don't recommend eating red meat every day, but if your body cries out for it, respond to those cries. It's a good idea to serve some kind of pickle with red meat, to **aid digestion. "**

2 x 125 g (4 oz) fillet steaks

1 tablespoon olive oil

2 servings Italian green salad
(page 27)

salsa

1 medium-sized vine-ripened tomato,
cut into small pieces

½ bunch fresh coriander (cilantro),
roughly chopped

½ small red chilli, seeded and
finely chopped

juice of 1 lime

½ cup kalamata olives, pitted
and finely chopped

½ tablespoon capers, rinsed
and chopped

serves 2

Wipe the fillet steaks with damp paper towel, brush with the olive oil and set aside at room temperature for no more than an hour. Combine the salsa ingredients in a bowl. Heat a barbecue or chargrill pan and add the steaks, cooking for 3–5 minutes on each side (according to your preference). Top each steak with salsa and serve with Italian green salad.

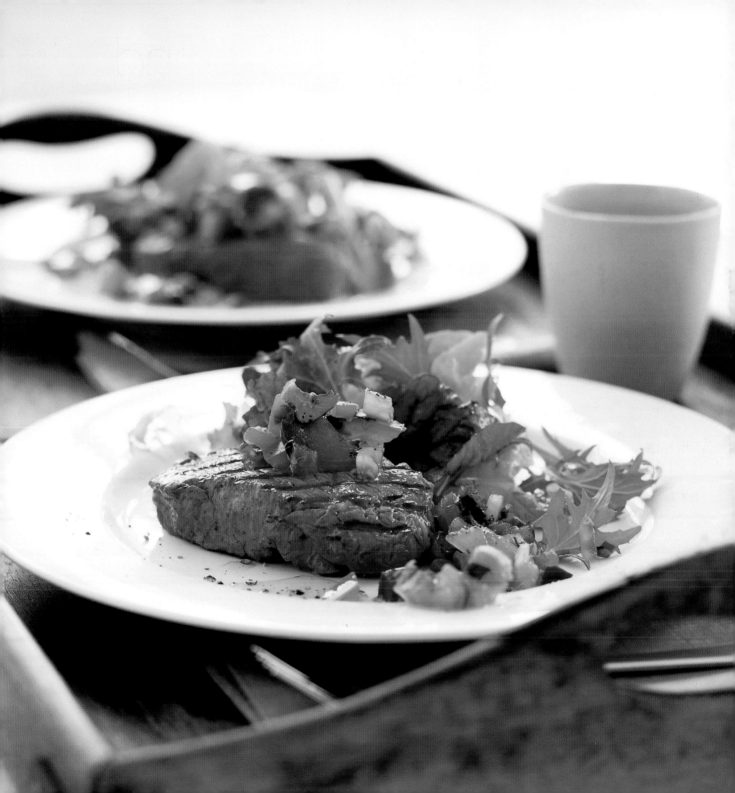

As with the breakfasts in this book, this collection of sweet treats uses grains, fruit and nuts, sweetened with honey, rice syrup, maple syrup, barley malt and fruit concentrates. Every now and then it's nice to have something sweet – and these are all relatively guilt-free. The sugars they contain tend to be absorbed less quickly than the refined sugar found in sweets. And while nuts are high in fat, it is a healthy type of fat.

Years ago (at the risk of making myself sound like a geriatric) women used to bake maybe once a week. When the tins were laden there were delicious sweet goodies to eat and, once these were gone, families would have to wait until the next baking day. Sweet biscuits (cookies) and cakes were considered treats.

It's too easy now to buy a selection of cakes and biscuits to have on hand every day. As a result, we eat too much and probably don't appreciate them as much as we could. I hope you enjoy these recipes, but hope even more that in the course of leading a healthier life through good food, your need for sweet things diminishes.

sweet treats

fresh pineapple with mint and coconut salsa

" There are times when you feel you have to serve a dessert – particularly when guests are coming over for dinner. This one is very easy and, if you want to indulge your guests, it would be nice served with a sorbet ice-cream. Pineapple contains an enzyme called bromelain, which **aids the digestive process**. Make sure the pineapple is ripe and sweet, otherwise it can be too acidic and cause stomach pain. **"**

1 small ripe pineapple

salsa

1 tablespoon maple syrup

juice of 1 lime

1 cup fresh mint, finely chopped

⅓ cup coconut flakes

serves 4

Peel the pineapple, cut into chunks and put in the fridge to chill. To make the salsa, combine the maple syrup and lime juice, then mix in the mint and coconut flakes. Spoon the salsa over the chilled pineapple.

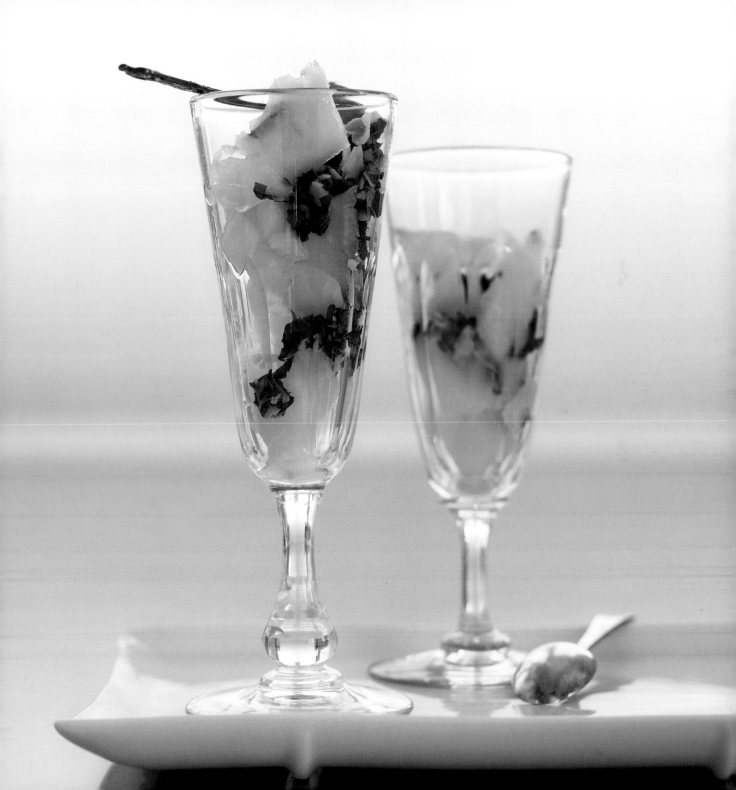

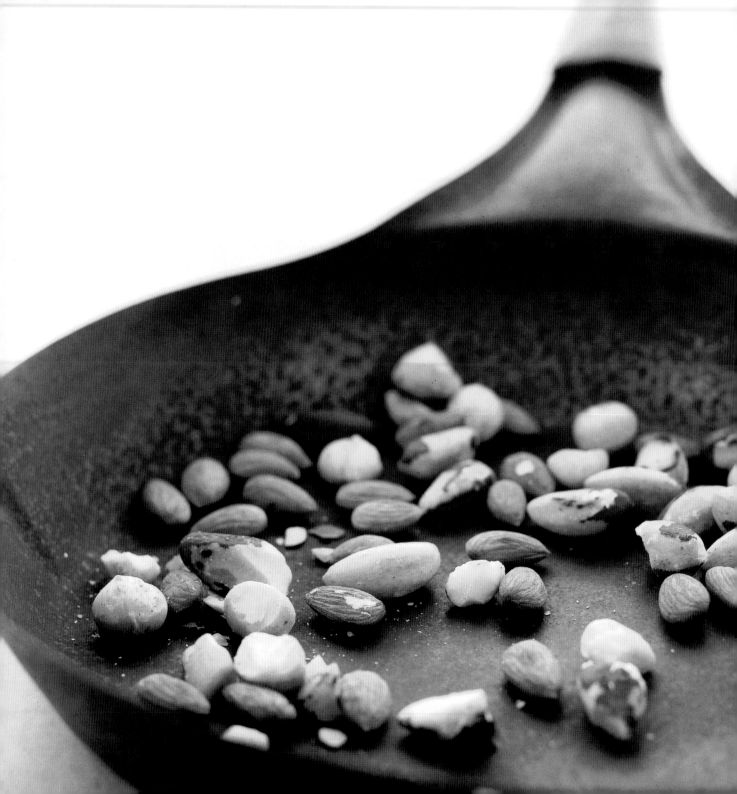

coconut energy bars

"This recipe was **written for one of my clients** who introduced a coconut chocolate bar into days 16 and 17 of her program (she ate the bar over two days). I hoped it was a craving for coconut that led her to it! Although I don't recommend that coconut is eaten too frequently, as it contains saturated fats, now and again it's fine. These bars are a little tricky to shape, but persevere – they are delicious. **"**

2 cups sunflower seeds

1 cup sesame seeds

1 cup almonds, chopped

¼ cup coconut flakes

½ cup dried apricots

½ cup sultanas

1½ cups rice syrup

makes about 20 squares

Separately dry-roast the sunflower and sesame seeds, almonds and coconut until toasted and fragrant. While these dry ingredients are still hot, mix in the dried fruit and rice syrup. Shape the mixture into a block while still warm. Once it is cool and has set, cut into small squares. Store in an airtight container in the pantry.

baked apples

"In winter, when large green Granny Smith apples are in season, there is no nicer way to end a meal than with these baked apples. The stuffing tastes a little like halva. This recipe is a variation on one that Karla Maverick, my macrobiotic cooking teacher, gave me."

¼ cup dates, finely chopped

¼ cup almonds, finely chopped

3 tablespoons hulled tahini

4 apples, cored

4 tablespoons soy milk

4 teaspoons rice syrup

serves 4

Preheat the oven to 180°C (350°F, Gas Mark 4). Mix the dates, almonds and tahini together in a bowl. Place each apple on a separate piece of foil and gently stuff with the tahini mixture. Carefully pour 1 tablespoon of the soy milk and 1 teaspoon of the rice syrup around the base of each apple then wrap in the foil. Place in a baking dish and bake for 35 minutes. Remove the foil and serve.

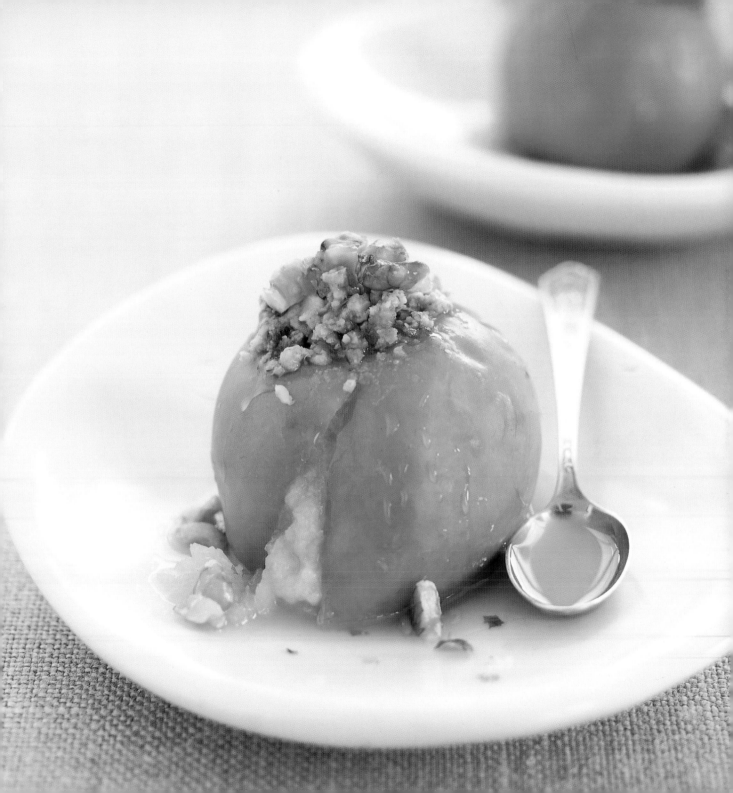

nut and fruit loaf

" This recipe came from a lady I met in a cafe one day. She was very distressed because her daughter had just been diagnosed with breast cancer for the second time. Over the years, through reading and research, she had learnt that soy can play a role in the **prevention of cancer**. It may be foolish to have too much faith that food could cure something as serious as cancer, but as food plays a huge role in preventing illness, it would be just as foolish not to try.

This loaf is packed full of nutritious goodies. It's a great fix for a sweet attack and incredibly easy, but prepare yourself – if you're expecting a light, fluffy-textured cake, you'll be in for a disappointment. It's heavy and tastes quite different from a normal fruit cake, but is equally enjoyable. It also makes a great breakfast toasted and served with ricotta cheese. "

2 cups soy milk

1 cup soy flour

1 cup organic wholemeal self-raising (self-rising) flour

1 cup rolled oats

¾ cup sultanas

¾ cup apricots, chopped

½ cup sesame seeds

½ cup sunflower seeds

½ cup slivered almonds

2 tablespoons grated fresh ginger

1 tablespoon barley malt (available at health food shops)

½ teaspoon ground cinnamon

½ teaspoon ground nutmeg

pinch sea salt

makes 1 medium-sized loaf

Preheat the oven to 190°C (375°F, Gas Mark 4) and line a loaf tin with baking paper, leaving sufficient paper on all sides to cover the top of the loaf tin. Mix all the ingredients together in a food processor. Fill the loaf tin with the mixture and cover with the overlapping paper. Refrigerate for 30 minutes then bake for 1 hour.

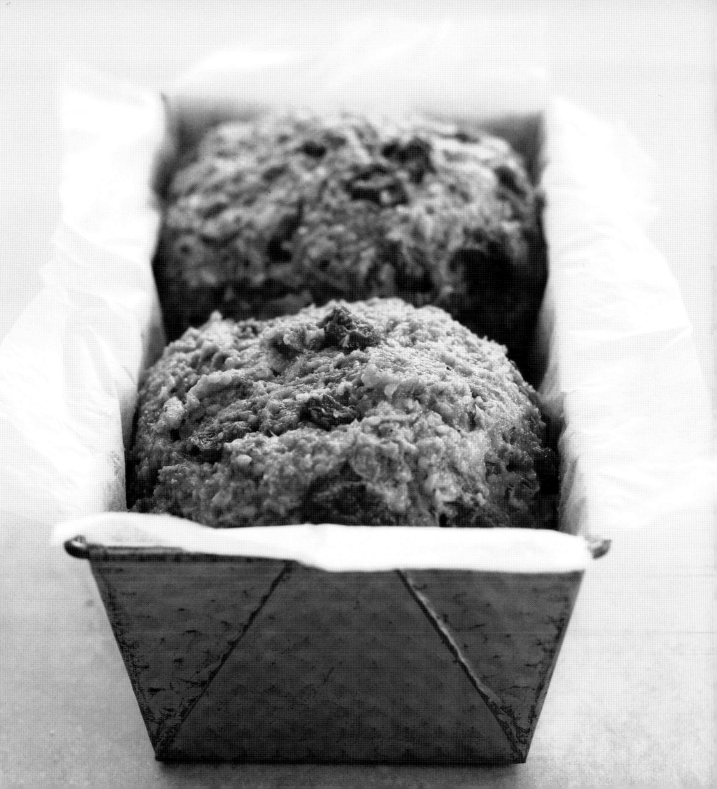

poached dried figs

" Many of us, particularly meat eaters, suffer from a mild form of acidosis – and figs are one of the most alkaline foods there is. I'm not sure that these figs poached in red wine will serve that well in relieving the symptoms of acidosis, but they are certainly not bad for you and, served with goat's cheese, oatcakes and strawberries, make a **perfect end to a dinner. "**

2 cups dried figs

2 cinnamon sticks

2 x 5 cm (2 in) strips orange peel

1 tablespoon orange zest

½ tablespoon maple syrup

about 1½ cups red wine

soft goat's cheese (chèvre), to serve

strawberries, to serve

Scottish oatcakes (page 56), to serve

serves 6

Place the figs, cinnamon sticks, orange peel, orange zest and maple syrup in a saucepan and pour over enough red wine to cover the figs. Slowly bring to the boil then reduce the heat to a simmer. Very slowly poach the figs for 1–1½ hours until they have absorbed the wine and are soft and surrounded by a thick syrup. Serve in a bowl, with the soft goat's cheese, strawberries and oatcakes on the side.

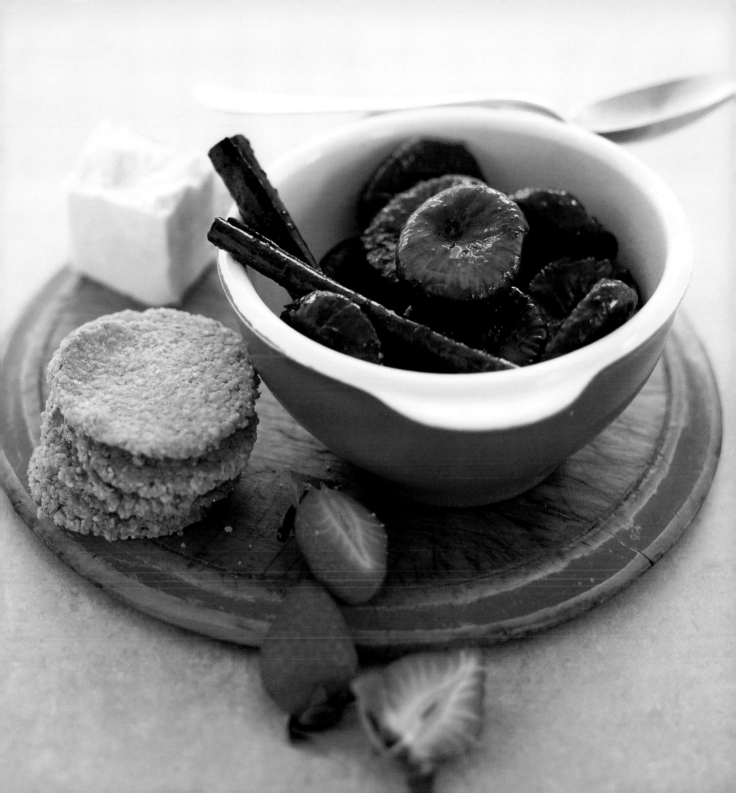

robert's biscuits

"Robert was one of my clients and **I'm rather proud to say** a devoted fan of 'The Food Coach'. He raved about my service to all who would listen, and followed my suggestions to the letter. His Achilles heel was the need for a sweet biscuit (cookie) with his cup of tea in the evening. He would experiment with baking on the weekends and even set his elderly mother to the task of inventing a healthy sweet biscuit 'with crunch'. To thank him for his support and friendship, I have included his recipe here – I invite you to try Robert's biscuits. **"**

⅓ cup honey

1⅓ cups coarse oatmeal

½ cup wholemeal plain
(all-purpose) flour

½ teaspoon bicarbonate of soda
(baking soda)

⅓ cup dried apricots, very finely
chopped

¼ cup slivered almonds

⅓ cup non-hydrogenated table spread

makes about 30 biscuits

Line a baking sheet with baking paper and preheat the oven to 160°C (325°F, Gas Mark 3). Gently heat the honey until it becomes very runny. In a food processor, mix together the oatmeal, flour, bicarbonate of soda, apricots and almonds. Add the table spread and process until the mixture resembles breadcrumbs, then add the honey. Mix briefly to form a firm dough then wrap in plastic and put in the freezer for 10–15 minutes. Using a rolling pin and a floured board, quickly roll out the dough to 5 mm (¼ in) thickness and cut into biscuits about 5 cm (2 in) in diameter. Bake for 15 minutes or until golden. Store in an airtight container in the pantry.

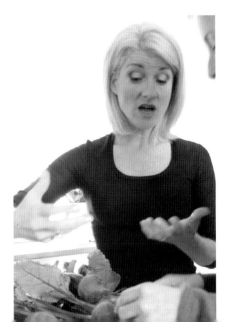

hedgehogs

"I know the name is awful, but I didn't want to put you off with the word 'carob'. Someone once told me that these little treats tasted like chocolate hedgehogs and, by the quantity she consumed, it seemed to be a positive thing. Imagine: it's Christmas Day in the UK, 'the feeding fest'. You've rolled away from the table to watch the Queen's speech over coffee (ask me now why I moved to Australia!). With coffee there is cream, Christmas cake, and other little chocolatey sweet things. Enter the hedgehogs. If you have a sweet tooth, *and* you like to eat healthily, you may prefer to **end your meal with these healthier alternatives** rather than abstain altogether. After all, it is Christmas Day and life is not about making sacrifices all the time.

Oh, and for the Harry Potter fans, don't attempt to make these unless you have the Nimbus 2000 food processor. For the rest of you, that means your food processor must be powerful."

2 cups rolled oats

1 cup dates

1 cup sultanas

½ cup almonds

2 tablespoons carob powder

1 teaspoon vanilla essence

makes about 24

Combine all the ingredients in a food processor until the mixture resembles fine breadcrumbs. Using your hands, mould the mixture into balls. Refrigerate for 30 minutes before serving. These hedgehogs can be stored in the fridge for up to 3 weeks.

rhubarb and ginger crumble

“ Feel free to replace the rhubarb with pears or any other fruit that works well in a crumble. The **topping is much healthier** than the traditional crumble made from flour, sugar and butter – and much nicer. ”

1 bunch rhubarb, trimmed

½ cup apple concentrate

1 teaspoon grated fresh ginger

¼ cup hazelnuts, dry-roasted

¼ cup almonds, dry-roasted

½ cup rolled oats, dry-roasted

¼ cup sunflower seeds, dry-roasted

¼ cup pumpkin seeds (pepitas),
  dry-roasted

1 tablespoon sesame seeds,
  dry-roasted

½ cup barley malt

1 tablespoon corn oil

¼ teaspoon ground cinnamon

serves 6

Preheat the oven to 160°C (325°F, Gas Mark 3). Wash the rhubarb but don't dry it, and cut into pieces about 2.5 cm (1 in) long. Put in a pan over a low heat, add the apple concentrate and ginger and cover. The rhubarb will slowly stew in the steam and its own juices. Remove from the heat when the rhubarb is tender but still retains its shape – about 5–10 minutes. Divide among 6 individual ramekins and set aside. Coarsely chop the roasted nuts and mix with the oats and seeds. Melt the barley malt in a saucepan with the corn oil and cinnamon and mix with a wooden spoon. Pour the oil and malt mixture over the nuts and mix until thoroughly combined. Spoon the crumble mixture over the rhubarb and bake for 15 minutes.

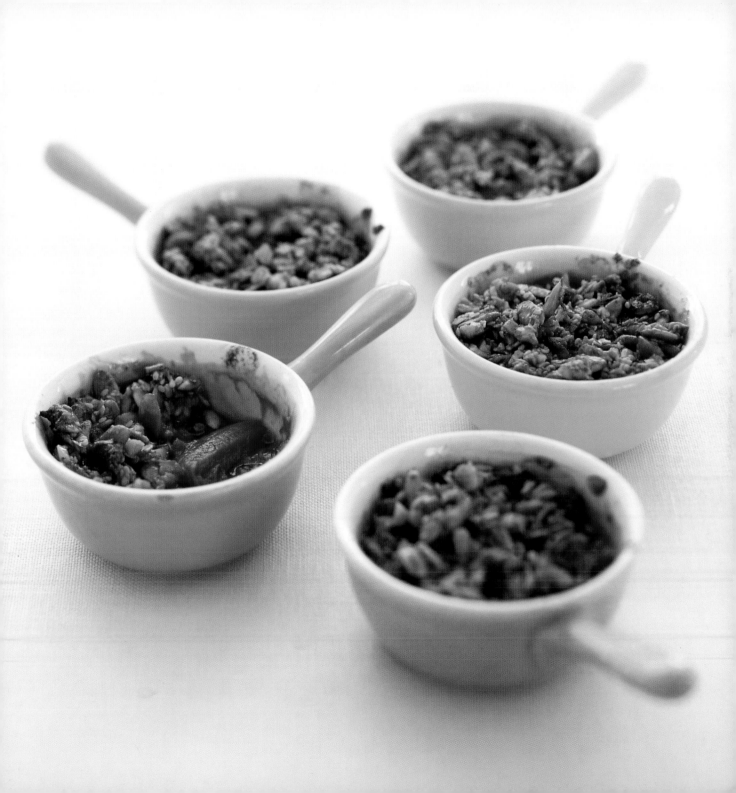

glossary of value-positive foods

BEETROOT (BEET) Beetroot contains folate, potassium and vitamin C – all essential for the maintenance of healthy cells. In Chinese medicine, beetroot is said to strengthen the heart, purify the blood, improve circulation, and cure liver ailments. For the Chinese, the liver is the 'General' that controls the actions of the other organs. If the liver is ailing it cannot adequately control its army of organs and, as a consequence, other health problems can arise. Beetroot leaves are often thrown out but steamed lightly they make a delicious, sweet-tasting salad rich in anti-oxidants, calcium and iron.

BERRIES Boysenberries, blueberries, cranberries, strawberries and raspberries are packed full of anti-oxidants. Raspberries and blueberries in particular are good sources of fibre and vitamin A and, according to the Chinese, excellent for cleansing the blood. As someone who insists on eating by the seasons, I make a hypocrite of myself by sometimes using frozen berries. Raspberries and blackberries freeze beautifully, retaining most of their nutritional value.

BONITO FLAKES Bonito flakes are dehydrated, thinly shaved fish flakes used to make dashi (Japanese stock). Available from Asian supermarkets, they are best bought in individual sachets.

BUCKWHEAT Buckwheat is gluten-free and can be used by people who suffer from cereal and grain allergies. Buckwheat noodles are a great substitute for pasta. They are higher in fibre, contain micronutrients that can help with vitamin C absorption, and impart a generally improved sense of wellbeing. The noodles take very little time to cook, an added bonus for anyone who is short of time. Buckwheat noodles can be bought from any Asian shop, some supermarkets and health food shops. The Japanese name for noodle is soba.

BURGHUL (BULGUR) Burghul is a type of wheat that can help stabilise blood sugar levels and keep us energised and calm throughout the day and night. It can be purchased from most health food stores and supermarkets.

DRIED APRICOTS Dried apricots are a source of iron, potassium and beta-carotene. Beta-carotene is a natural anti-oxidant that helps promote long-term good health and also helps combat ageing and disease.

GARLIC Garlic has antiviral and antibacterial properties and can be used to treat a multitude of ailments. It is also said to help lower blood pressure and reduce high levels of blood cholesterol.

GINGER Fresh ginger root in juices, stir-fries and cakes tastes sensational and has so much nutritional value. Ginger helps break down meat and other proteins to lessen the effect of acid build-up, which is caused by excess protein consumption. Ginger is also useful in the treatment of nausea, morning sickness, period cramps, travel sickness and bronchitis.

GOAT'S MILK AND GOAT'S CHEESE (CHÈVRE) Like yoghurt, goat's milk and goat's cheese can often be tolerated by those sensitive to lactose. Goat's milk is easier to digest than cow's milk and is nutritionally more valuable. People who suffer from migraines triggered by cheese are often unaffected by goat's cheese.

GRAINS Many people caught up on the low-GI bandwagon are cutting out bread and rice, but there are many other grain foods that should be included in the diet. I recommend grains at breakfast. Fibre in the diet is essential to sweep away toxins from the intestine lining, and breakfast grains provide a substantial amount of dietary fibre. The key is to eat whole grains, such as oats, barley and rye. Wholegrain sourdough is a good choice of bread, as it has a lower GI than wholemeal and many other breads. Brown rice has a relatively high GI, but as it contains more nutrients and fibre than white rice, it should still be included in the diet.

KOMBU, NORI AND OTHER SEA VEGETABLES Sea vegetables contain up to twenty times the minerals of land plants and a huge amount of vitamins. They are especially excellent sources of calcium, iodine and iron. An easy introduction to the fruits of the sea is kombu, which is very high in minerals and increases the nutritional value of all food. Its healing properties include strengthening the kidneys, relieving hormone imbalances, reducing swelling and soothing the lungs and throat. It can increase the digestibility of beans and is the base for Japanese stock (dashi).

KUDZU Kudzu is a natural thickener from Japan that soothes the stomach and intestines. It can be purchased from Asian supermarkets or most good health food shops.

LEGUMES Legumes are low in fat and high in fibre. They are a good source of protein for vegetarians (when combined with a grain), are rich in nutrients and have a low GI. Legumes are a source of carbohydrate for energy, protein for cell maintenance and fibre to aid elimination of toxins. Often neglected as a staple food by our modern, fast-paced society, they are surprisingly easy to prepare. Organic cooked legumes can now be bought in cans, so those who have ruled them out previously, declaring them to be too time-consuming, now have no excuse!

Most legumes (except lentils and split peas) require soaking overnight before they are cooked, to remove some toxic substances and to reduce flatulence. Soak in 3 cups of water for each cup of beans. Drain the soaked beans and put in a pan with the same amount of fresh water and a 5 cm (2 in) piece of kombu. Bring the water to the boil then reduce to a simmer (see below for suggested cooking times). Add a pinch of sea salt in the last 5 minutes of cooking. Once cooked, skim off any froth, which will also cause flatulence, and discard the kombu. One cup of dried beans will give you about 2 cups of cooked beans. Cooked beans can be frozen.

legume	cooking time
adzuki beans	1 hour
black beans	2 hours
cannellini beans	1–1½ hours
chickpeas (garbanzo beans)	1–1½ hours
green (Puy) lentils★	15–20 minutes

haricot (navy) beans	1 hour
kidney beans	1–1½ hours
lima (butter) beans	1–1½ hours
red lentils★	15 minutes
soybeans	1–4 hours

★ soaking not required

KUMARA (SWEET POTATO) Kumara is very high in vitamin A and can therefore help night vision. It has a lower GI than potatoes of any sort. Being sweet, kumara can help to curb the craving for sweet things after the main meal. For that reason I encourage people to eat kumara rather than potato or the similarly high-GI pumpkin (squash). Kumara also contains anti-oxidants.

LEMONS Lemons break down fats and proteins. The juice detoxifies the blood and encourages weight loss. Lemons are often used to ease chesty colds and sore throats, as they can help to break down mucus.

LINSEED (FLAX SEED) Flax seeds or linseeds are the richest plant source of omega-3 fatty acids, which strengthen the immune system and cleanse the heart and arteries.

MIRIN Mirin is a slightly sweet Japanese cooking sherry made from rice. It adds flavour to many Japanese dishes.

MISO Miso is a fermented soybean paste. It is high in salt, so use in moderation, but it gives a wonderful flavour to soups, stews and dressings. It is said to promote long life and good health. Miso, like yoghurt with *Acidophilus*, aids digestion and helps strengthen the immune system, but if it is boiled for over a minute its healing properties are destroyed. Buy miso paste from a health food shop or Asian supermarket; it will keep for months in the fridge.

MOONFISH (OPAH) Moonfish is used frequently by the Chinese community. A by-catch of tuna, it is rich in similar nutrients and is a good source of omega-3 fatty acids.

MUSHROOMS Mushrooms are high in fibre and a rich source of magnesium, phosphorus, selenium and potassium. They help maintain strong teeth and bones, protect the muscular and nervous systems and fight harmful free radicals. Mushrooms are also thought to help remove mucus on the chest and boost the immune system. When preparing mushrooms, either peel the skin off or wipe off any dirt with a soft brush – don't wash them. Store mushrooms in a paper bag in the fridge, but never store them in plastic, or they sweat and become slimy.

NATURAL YOGHURT Natural yoghurt is a natural antibiotic that helps stimulate the immune system to fight viruses and infection. It contains live cultures that promote the growth of healthy bacteria in the intestine. It is an excellent source of calcium, phosphorus and some B vitamins. During the making of yoghurt, lactose is broken down, making it a useful source of calcium for people who suffer from lactose intolerance or who otherwise do not eat dairy. Buy low-fat yoghurt with added *Acidophilus*.

NUTS AND SEEDS While nuts are high in fat, it is considered to be 'good fat'. Most nuts are rich sources of nutrients and should be included in the diet (provided there is no allergy). Nuts can become rancid if old and not stored properly; check the expiry date on all nuts and store them in ⬚⬚⬚⬚⬚ Rancid nuts are hazardous to the body, causing production of free radicals, ⬚⬚⬚⬚⬚ nge of health problems, including cancer and other chronic diseases.

Almonds are considere⬚⬚⬚⬚⬚ he stomach digests food it releases very acidic enzymes, which can cause a ⬚⬚⬚⬚⬚ isorders and joint pain (particularly common in those with diets high in red⬚⬚⬚⬚⬚ elp alkalise the blood, reducing the effects of these acidic enzymes. They ar⬚⬚⬚⬚⬚ cium.

Brazil nuts are rich in se⬚⬚⬚⬚⬚ a day will ward off prostate cancer. Selenium is an anti-oxidant that helps str⬚⬚⬚⬚⬚ It is also said to be a natural antidepressant. *Peanuts* are legumes that grow ⬚⬚⬚⬚⬚ ery low GI. As peanuts absorb toxins from the soil it is advisable always to ⬚⬚⬚⬚⬚

Pine nuts are the richest s⬚⬚⬚⬚⬚ Mediterranean and in the East they are also reputed to have aphrodisiac prop⬚⬚⬚⬚⬚ and zinc. They can alleviate pain, reduce inflammation and ease stress, and ⬚⬚⬚⬚⬚ ease.

Pumpkin seeds are a good ⬚⬚⬚⬚⬚ fatty acids. While not as high in fibre as sunflower and sesame seeds, they ⬚⬚⬚⬚⬚ ood source of protein, calcium, zinc and vitamin E. They are high in unsat⬚⬚⬚⬚⬚ levels. They are high in fibre and impart a delicious nutty flavour to salads ⬚⬚⬚⬚⬚ the fridge to prevent rancidity. *Sunflower seeds* are high in linoleic acid, whic⬚⬚⬚⬚⬚ n in fibre and vitamin E. *Nigella seeds* are said to help hay fever, headaches, ha⬚⬚⬚⬚⬚

OATS Go for organic rolled oats ra⬚⬚⬚⬚⬚ . Oats are a good source of protein, B vitamins, calcium and fibre. They h⬚⬚⬚⬚⬚ he few grains that do not have the bran and germ removed during processir⬚⬚⬚⬚⬚ (sometimes called pin-head oatmeal), which have a lower GI and make the⬚⬚⬚⬚⬚

OLIVE OIL Never be without a bottl⬚⬚⬚⬚⬚ oil helps lower 'bad' cholesterol and decrease the risk of heart disease. It is⬚⬚⬚⬚⬚ ght disease and premature ageing.

PARSLEY Both types of parsley – flat⬚⬚⬚⬚⬚ ully good for you, although flat-leaf parsley is usually preferred for its textu⬚⬚⬚⬚⬚ in plentiful amounts; it's loaded with vitamins A and C, calcium, iron, potass⬚⬚⬚⬚⬚

POLENTA (CORNMEAL) Polenta is coarsely⬚⬚⬚⬚⬚ , a soft, comforting carbohydrate that can help stimulate an appetite depleted th⬚⬚⬚⬚⬚ s high in vitamin A. Use it as a substitute for breadcrumbs if wheat-intolerant.⬚⬚⬚⬚⬚ nake pancakes and breakfast cereals.

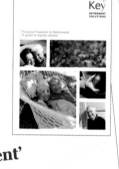

PRUNES Prunes are a good source of potassium, iron, vitamin B$_6$ and fibre. Like other dried foods, they have a high sugar content and should be eaten in moderation.

RHUBARB Surprisingly, rhubarb is an excellent source of calcium, one cup providing almost half the calcium of the same amount of whole milk. In Chinese medicine, rhubarb is used to detoxify the liver. As it is extremely tart, most people negate any beneficial properties by cooking it in mountainous amounts of sugar. Stew rhubarb with pears and a tablespoon of pear concentrate to take the edge off this delicious vegetable.

RICE SYRUP Rice syrup is made from fermented rice grain and can be purchased from any health food shop. It is a better choice of sweetener than sugar, as it takes longer to digest than commercial white sugars and therefore helps to regulate blood sugar peaks and troughs.

RICE VINEGAR This delicately flavoured, naturally brewed vinegar is made from fermented brown rice. Rice vinegar and apple cider vinegar contain minerals that have a detoxifying effect on the liver.

SEA SALT Salt has gained a reputation as the number one enemy of good health, but most research on salt and its contribution to chronic disease is based on refined salt, which contains many chemicals, including anti-caking agents, potassium iodide and sugar. While there is absolutely no doubt that too much salt is harmful, a good-quality sea salt used sparingly in cooking can strengthen the digestion and help neutralise acid conditions in the body.

SHIITAKE MUSHROOMS This gem of a mushroom is said to help lower fat and cholesterol levels in the blood and contains compounds that induce an immune response against cancer and viral disease.

SHOYU (SOY SAUCE) Shoyu or soy sauce is traditionally made from wheat, soybeans, water and sea salt. Take the time to read the label; some commercial soy sauces contain caramel and other additives.

TAHINI Tahini is a paste made from hulled or unhulled sesame seeds. Unhulled tahini is much darker and is higher in fibre. Use it on toast instead of butter and in dips and spreads.

TAMARI Tamari is a wheat-free seasoning made from the liquid extract obtained during the making of miso from soybeans. It is suitable for people with wheat allergies. Tamari tastes similar to shoyu, but sharper.

THYME Thyme is said to be useful if you need to treat parasites in the stomach. Thyme tea relieves indigestion, lifts the spirits and relieves the symptoms of colds, bronchitis and sinusitis.

TOFU Tofu is a brilliant blank canvas and can assume any flavour. Excellent for vegetarians, it is a complete source of protein, low in calories, contains no cholesterol or saturated fat and is packed full of vitamins and minerals, including vitamin B, calcium and iron. To flavour firm tofu, boil it in water until it floats to the surface, then drain and blot dry with absorbent paper. Firm tofu is good for stir-fries and snacks, while silken tofu can be used in desserts. Once you have opened a packet of tofu, store any leftovers covered with water in a plastic container in the fridge. Replace the water every day and the tofu will keep for about five days.

index

acknowledgements

The criteria for the recipes in this book were they had to be healthy, delicious and easy. They also had to work. Without my 'testers', the recipes may not have met these requirements. I would like to thank my friends and past clients who volunteered their time (and tastebuds) to test these recipes and help me decide which stayed and which went. Some of these testers were chosen because they stick to a recipe (I never do), others because they lead healthy lives and embrace my philosophy, and the rest because I had to challenge their beliefs and prove that healthy food can be delicious. The following wonderful people were my testers: my sister, Jennifer Aveyard; John Serafini and Craig Glasson; Robert Hall and Mark Hampson; Melinda and Greg Wilson; Des Doyle and Jill Livesey; Tracey and Brett Jordan; Kirsty Simmonds; Lorraine Brooks; Anne Bottomley and Madison Parker; Marsha Marsh; and Jennifer Nielsen.

Thanks also to Macro Wholefoods, Claudio's Seafoods, Clover Foods and Gourmet Cuisine, who supplied many of the ingredients shown in the photographs, and to Atmosphere in Surry Hills, Stem in Balmain, Plenty in Balmain and Essential in Randwick for generously lending some of the homewares that appear in the photographs.

Special thanks to Bill Tikos, my agent, without whom this book may never have been written, and to Julie Gibbs from Penguin, who saw my potential and was prepared to take a risk and publish this, my first book.

Finally, lashings and lashings of love and thanks to the team who made this book a reality; at the start of the project I was humbled to be working with such talent and experience. John Paul Urizar's food photography makes people buy books – that's probably why you are reading this one! Julz Beresford, food stylist, makes everything look amazing on a plate. My lovely friend Michelle Rickerby quietly and calmly supported me in the kitchen and anticipated my every need. Nicola Young edited all my terrible mistakes and taught me how to use the comma, and Penguin's award-winning designer Melissa Fraser created this beautiful design. Thanks also to Lucy Baldock, the talented make-up artist, and, of course, to Boots the dog. It was humbling and moving to work with such lovely people who were all genuinely committed to making this book the best it could be, and who at the end of this project I call my friends.